Workbook for

Health Careers Today

Workbook for

Health Careers Today

Fifth Edition

Judith Gerdin, BSN, MS
Phoenix, Arizona

ELSEVIER
MOSBY

3251 Riverport Lane
St. Louis, Missouri 63043

WORKBOOK FOR HEALTH CAREERS TODAY, 5TH EDITION   ISBN: 978-0-323-07995-2

ISBN: 978-0-323-07995-2

Publishing Director: Andrew Allen
Managing Editor: Ellen Wurm-Cutter
Developmental Editor: Kristen Mandava
Publishing Services Manager: Julie Eddy/Anitha Raj
Project Managers: Sukanthi Sukumar/Jan Waters
Designer: Amy Buxton

Printed in the United States of America

Last digit is the print number: 9   8   7   6   5   4   3

Preface to the Student

This workbook was designed for use with the textbook *Health Careers Today*. It provides exercises that reinforce the information presented in the textbook and activities that allow you, the student, to demonstrate that material. With the new section, Internet Activities, you will have the opportunity to enlarge upon and personalize the information provided in the textbook.

The chapters of the workbook are divided into the following sections:

- Vapid Vocabulary—provides puzzles that review the key terms of each chapter.
- Abbreviations—presents 10 medical abbreviations that are included in the content of the chapter.
- Just the Facts—uses fill-in-the-blank sentences to test your recall of factual information presented in the chapter.
- Concept Applications—allows you to review and use information from the chapter.
- Investigations—provides laboratory exercises that apply and expand on the information provided in the textbook. These activities should be completed under the supervision of a qualified professional only.
- Critical Thinking Exercises—develops your awareness of health care concerns and expands your thinking skills. These exercises often ask for your opinion and may have more than one correct answer.
- Internet Activities—allows you to explore the most current and personally relevant information available, using the suggested links and individualized Internet research.

Your teacher will give you directions regarding which of these components you are to complete to meet the objectives of your class.

Judith A. Gerdin

Contents

VAPID VOCABULARY

Complete the crossword puzzle using the Key Terms.

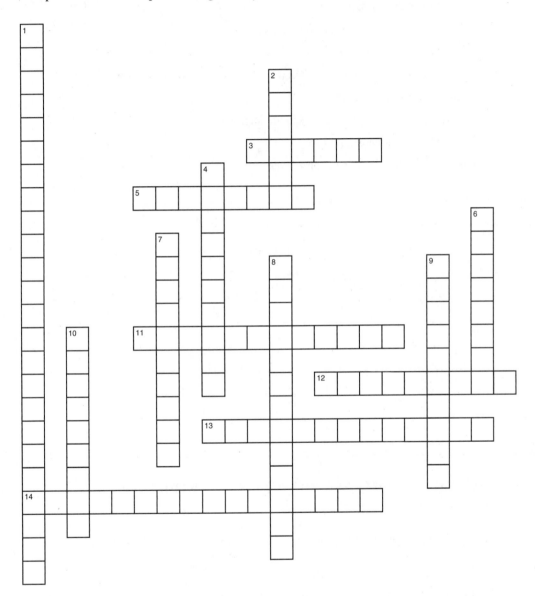

ACROSS

3 State of optimal well-being, achieved through prevention of illness and injury
5 Treatment that pretends to cure disease
11 Official record of individuals qualified to perform certain services
12 Payment for health care expenses, which may or may not occur, in return for a specified payment in advance
13 Documentation of having met certain standards
14 Worker who assists a professional in the performance of duties

DOWN

1 Predetermined payment structure for health care services established by the federal government (three words)
2 Occupation or profession
4 Vocation, activity in which one participates
6 Epidemic that spreads over a wide geographical area, affecting a large part of the population
7 Occupation that requires specialized knowledge and, often, long and intensive academic training
8 Official authorization or approval
9 Legal dispute; lawsuit
10 Legal authority to perform an activity

ABBREVIATIONS

Match each of the following abbreviations with the phrase that best describes its meaning or function. Then write the phrase or name for each of the abbreviations in the spaces that follow.

Abbreviation	Meaning or Function
1. _____ CDC	a. Agency responsible for safety of drugs
2. _____ DRG	b. Agency that monitors and prevents outbreaks of disease
3. _____ FDA	c. Communicable disease
4. _____ GDP	d. Health care costs represent over 16% of this
5. _____ HHS	e. Managed health care
6. _____ HMO	f. Members are allowed to select treatment for in or out of the network
7. _____ NIH	g. Provides research money
8. _____ POS	h. Reimbursement for services based on diagnosis
9. _____ PPO	i. Represents national health care
10. _____ TB	j. Selected health care agency or worker

1. CDC: _____

2. DRG: _____

3. FDA: _____

4. GDP: _____

5. HHS: _____

6. HMO: _____

7. NIH: _____

8. POS: _____

9. PPO: _____

10. TB: _____

JUST THE FACTS

1. Some medications in current use come from herbs and plants that were used in the past, including

   _ _ _ _O_ _ _ _ and _ _ _ _ _ _O_ _ _ _.

2. The focus of health care has shifted from the prevention of contagious diseases to those that are related to lifestyle choices, such as _ _ _O_ _ _ _, _ _ _ _ _ _ _ _ _ _ _, and _O_ _ _ _ _disease.

3. The agency of the federal government that oversees the nation's health care is the _ _ _ _ _ _ _ _ _O_ _ _ _ _ _ _ _ _ _O_ _.

4. Some of the influences on health care in the United States include the state of the _ _O_ _ _ _ _ _, the law of supply and _ _ _O_ _ _, and _ _ _ _ _ _ _ _O_ _.

5. Some of the opportunities that are provided to health care workers include new _ _ _ _O_ _ _ _ _ _, a stable _ _ _ _ _ _ and employment, and the ability to move to new locations.

6. The credentials that may be required for employment in the health care industry include

_ _ _ Ⓞ _ _ _ _ _ , _ _ _ Ⓞ _ _ _ _ _ _ _ _ _ _ _ , and

_ _ _ _ _ _ _ _ _ _ Ⓞ _ _ _.

7. One of the influences that will affect health care in the future is the growing population of

_ _ _ _ _ _ _.

8. Innovations that will affect health care of the future include

_ Ⓞ _ _ _ _ _ _ _ Ⓞ _ _ _ _ _ and telemedicine.

9. The Internet provides information about Ⓞ _ _ _ _ _ _ Ⓞ _ _ _ _ _ _ _ _ _

that may not be from a reputable practitioner.

10. Health care workers of the future must be _ Ⓞ _ _ _ _ _ _, able to solve

_ Ⓞ _ _ _ _ _ _, and willing to continue to _ Ⓞ _ _ _.

Use the circled letters to form the answer to this jumble. Clue: Until 2010, what was one characteristic of the United States that separated it from all other industrial nations?

_ _   _ _ _ _ _ _ _   _ _ _ _ _ _ _ _ _

CONCEPT APPLICATIONS

Historical Perspectives
Choose 10 of the milestones of health care progress from the Medical Milestones box at the end of Chapter 1 in the textbook to construct a time line of health care progress in Figure 1-1.

Figure 1-1

Trends of Today
Using the local newspaper or online resources, determine which health career positions are available in the local area. Use your observations to answer the following questions.

1. Which job category has the most advertisements for unfilled job opportunities?

_____

_____

_____

2. Use the textbook to write a description of the job duties of the position you identified in question 1.

_____

_____

_____

3. Why do you think there is such a high demand for the career you identified in question 1?

_____

_____

_____

Chapter **1** **Health Care of the Past, Present, and Future**

4. Relate to this occupation one of the medical milestones found in the box at the end of Chapter 1 in the textbook.

_____

_____

_____

CAREERS OF THE FUTURE

According to studies by the U.S. Department of Labor, the fastest-growing occupations or those projected to have the largest numerical increases in employment between 2006 and 2016 include those listed as follows.

Use the textbook and the Internet to describe the job duties of three of the occupations listed.

OCCUPATION	% INCREASE	EDUCATION
Personal and home care aides	50.6	Short-term and on-the-job training
Home health aides	48.7	Short-term and on-the-job training
Veterinary technologist and technicians	41.0	Associate degree
Medical assistant	35.4	Moderate-term and on-the-job training
Veterinarian	35.0	First professional degree
Substance abuse and behavioral disorder counselor	34.3	Bachelor's degree
Social and human service assistant	33.6	Moderate-term and on-the-job training
Physical therapist assistant	32.4	Associate degree
Pharmacy technician	32.0	Moderate-term and on-the-job training
Forensic science technician	30.7	Bachelor's degree
Dental hygienist	30.1	Associate degree
Mental health counselor	30.0	Master's degree
Mental health and substance abuse social worker	29.9	Master's degree
Marriage and family therapist	29.8	Master's degree
Dental assistant	29.2	Moderate-term and on-the-job training
Environmental science and protection technicians, including health	28.0	Associate degree
Physical therapist	27.1	Master's degree
Physician assistant	27.0	Master's degree

1. Career: _____

   Job duties: _____

   _____

   _____

2. Career: _____

   Job duties: _____

   _____

   _____

Chapter **1** **Health Care of the Past, Present, and Future**

3. Career: _____

   Job duties: _____

   _____

   _____

CRITICAL THINKING

Reducing the Threat of Disease

In 2006, the CDC reported the following conditions as the top 10 causes of death in the United States:

- Heart disease: 631,636
- Cancer: 559,888
- Stroke (cerebrovascular diseases): 137,119
- Chronic lower respiratory diseases: 124,583
- Accidents (unintentional injuries): 121,599
- Diabetes: 72,449
- Alzheimer's disease: 72,432
- Influenza and pneumonia: 56,326
- Nephritis, nephrotic syndrome, and nephrosis: 45,344
- Septicemia: 34,234

They can all be influenced significantly by nutrition, exercise, and the use of safety precautions.

Choose three conditions from the list and suggest one lifestyle change that would reduce the risk of developing it. Suggest one excuse that a person might use when choosing not to make the change.

Create a brochure describing one of the conditions, its consequences, and the lifestyle changes that would prevent it.

1. Condition: _____

   Lifestyle change: _____

   Excuse for not changing: _____

2. Condition: _____

   Lifestyle change: _____

   Excuse for not changing: _____

3. Condition: _____

   Lifestyle change: _____

   Excuse for not changing: _____

THE COST OF HEALTH CARE

The American Medical Association estimates that 15% of all medical costs result from what is called "defensive medicine," or testing designed to prevent malpractice suits. According to a study by the Massachusetts Medical Society and the University of Connecticut Health Center, the practice of defensive medicine is widespread. Defensive medicine includes tests, procedures, referrals, hospitalization, and prescriptions that are ordered because of fear of a possible lawsuit. In Massachusetts, these practices cost a minimum of $1.4 billion per year.

Some suggestions that have been proposed to reduce unnecessary expenditures include:

- Limiting the liability of the medical doctor in the case of misdiagnosis
- Establishing guidelines for signs and symptoms that require further testing
- Providing insurance reimbursement only for tests commonly used for given specific signs and symptoms

Answer the following questions regarding methods to reduce health care costs.

1. Propose at least one more method that might be used to reduce the number of unnecessary tests performed.

_____

_____

2. Examine each proposal, and explain why you believe it would or would not reduce the number of unnecessary tests.

   a. Limiting medical liability

   _____

   _____

   b. Establishing guidelines for necessary tests

   _____

   _____

   c. Limiting reimbursement for tests

   _____

   _____

3. Discuss the possibility of cost containment in one other area of health care.

   _____

   _____

   _____

INTERNET INVESTIGATIONS

Doctors Without Borders

Use the Internet links that follow to write an essay that describes the work of Doctors Without Borders and the study of SARS. Include the following information:
- What Doctors Without Borders is
- What SARS is
- When and where the first outbreak of SARS occurred
- What health personnel were involved in the investigation of the first outbreak
- How the deaths of the medical personnel, such as Carlo Urbani, occurred

Doctors Without Borders: http://doctorswithoutborders.org/
CDC Patient Treatment Hemorrhagic Fever: http://www.cdc.gov/mmwr/preview/mmwrhtml/00038033.htm
WHO—Urbani: http://www.who.int/csr/sars/urbani/en/
The New England Journal of Medicine—Urbani: http://content.nejm.org/cgi/content/full/348/20/1951

Medical Milestones

Use the Internet to research and answer the following questions.

1. What is the *placebo effect*?

   _____

   _____

2. List five examples of animal parts and minerals that were used in the past by primitive physicians.

   _____

   _____

6

3. Who was Galen and on what were his principles based?

_____

_____

4. Why was a surgeon considered to be of a lower status than a physician during the Renaissance?

_____

_____

5. When did federal controls over the drug supply begin in the United States?

_____

6. What is the most popular drug of all time?

_____

7. What were the two reasons for the passage of the Food and Drug Act of 1906?

_____

_____

8. When was penicillin discovered?

_____

9. When was the first test-tube baby born?

_____

10. When did scientists first clone sheep?

_____

_____

VAPID VOCABULARY

Complete the crossword puzzle using the Key Terms.

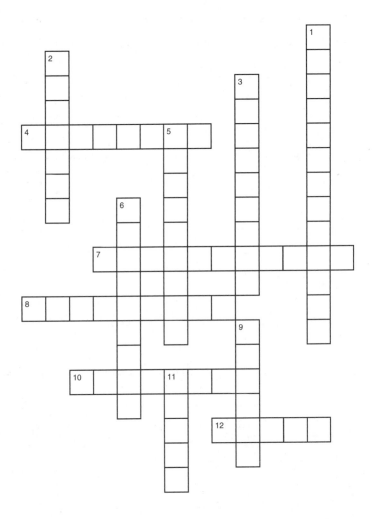

ACROSS

4 Mental position or feeling with regard to a fact or situation
7 Set of traits, characteristics, and behaviors that make each person unique
8 Distinctive qualities that make up an individual
10 Manner of conducting oneself
12 Act performed voluntarily without conscious thought

DOWN

1 Exchange of information
2 Sum of the socially gained patterns that guide a person's way of life, including values, beliefs, language, and thought
3 Communicating without using language
5 Quality of being different
6 Graded or ranked series
9 Relating to or consisting of words or sounds
11 Rate of usefulness, importance, or general worth

ABBREVIATIONS

Match each of the following abbreviations with the phrase that best describes its meaning or function. Then write the phrase or name for each of the abbreviations in the spaces.

Abbreviation	Meaning or Function
1. _____ cc	a. Electronic device used to collect patient information
2. _____ EMR	b. Electronic information or chart
3. _____ FPO	c. Federal law protecting confidentiality of patient information
4. _____ HIPAA	d. Health care worker responsible for daily care of patients
5. _____ I & O	e. Health care worker responsible for writing orders that direct the care of patients
6. _____ MD	f. Health care worker who determines what patient information can be shared
7. _____ NA	g. Record of fluids taken in and out of a patient
8. _____ PHI	h. Sensitive issues about a patient
9. _____ PDA	i. Team leader of health care workers
10. _____ RN	j. Unit of fluid

1. cc: _____

2. EMR: _____

3. FPO: _____

4. HIPAA: _____

5. I & O: _____

6. MD: _____

7. NA: _____

8. PHI: _____

9. PDA: _____

10. RN: _____

JUST THE FACTS

1. Health care workers must be able to communicate _ _ _ _ _ _ _ _ _ _ _ _ _, provide _ _ _ _ _ _ _ _ _ _ _, and use _ _ _ _ _ _ _ _ _ _ _ _ _ _ equipment.

2. Some skills helpful in interpersonal relationships include communicating _ _ _ _, acting _ _ _ _ _ _ _ _ _ _ _ _ _ _, and demonstrating _ _ _ _ _ _ _ _ _ _ _.

3. How a person thinks determines his or her _ _ _ _ _ _ _ _ and _ _ _ _ _ _ _ _ _ _ that result from an event.

4. Character is the sum of the _ _ _ _ _ _ _ _, attitudes, and _ _ _ _ _ _ that a person shows to others.

5. The World Health Organization defines health as a state of _ _ _ _ _ _ _ _, _ _ _ _ _ _, and social well-being.

Chapter **2** **Interpersonal Dynamics and Communications**

6. Many diseases cause symptoms of general stress, including fatigue, weight loss, aches, and
_ _ _ _ _ _ _ ◯ _ _ ◯ _ _ _ _ _ _ problems.

7. Stress may be managed with proper ◯ _ _ _ _ _ _ _ _ ◯, _ _ _ ◯ _ _ _ _,
_ _ _ _ ◯ _ _ _ _ _ techniques, and changes in personal behavior.

8. Critical thinking includes intentional application of _ _ ◯ _ _ ◯ _ _, higher-order thinking skills.

9. Assertive communication allows each person to express feelings, opinions, and beliefs in a
_ _ _ _ ◯◯ _ _ _ _ and _ _ _ _ ◯ _ _ _ _ _ ◯ manner.

10. With effective communication, the _ _ _ _ _ _ and ◯ _ _ _ _ _ _ _ _ _
messages are the same.

Use the circled letters to form the answer to this jumble. Clue: On what foundation is a person's value system formed?

_ _

CONCEPT APPLICATIONS

Personal Grooming Checklist
Good grooming habits are essential in all areas of health care. Take this short survey to evaluate your personal grooming habits. Identify three areas of personal grooming that you would like to improve. Chart in the spaces provided your effort to improve one of the three habits over the next 4 weeks.

YES	NO	GROOMING OR HEALTH HABIT
		I maintain my health by seeing a doctor when necessary.
		I maintain my health by eating a well-balanced diet.
		I maintain my health by using good posture.
		I bathe or shower every day.
		I shampoo my hair regularly.
		I keep my hair styled in a neat manner (away from my face and off of my collar).
		I use deodorant every day.
		I maintain my skin by using lotion and treating skin disorders as needed.
		I shave daily (men) or as needed (women) to remove unsightly hair.
		I wear clean undergarments daily.
		I wear all appropriate undergarments.
		I brush my teeth regularly (at least twice daily).
		I floss my teeth regularly (at least once daily).
		I use mouthwash regularly (at least once daily).
		I visit the dentist at least once yearly.
		I keep my fingernails clean and trimmed evenly.

Continued

Chapter **2** **Interpersonal Dynamics and Communications**

YES	NO	GROOMING OR HEALTH HABIT
		I wear clothes that fit properly.
		I wear clothes that are clean and pressed.
		I keep my clothes mended.
		I change my socks or stockings daily to reduce foot odor.
		I wear shoes that are clean and fit properly.
		I wear a clean uniform each day, which includes my name tag, watch, black pen, and writing paper.
		I wear shoes with my uniform that are nonskid, sturdy, and have low heels.
		I wear minimal jewelry with my uniform.
		I wear no perfume or cologne with my uniform to avoid irritating clients who are ill.

List three ways you can improve your personal health or grooming.

1. _____
_____
_____

2. _____
_____
_____

3. _____
_____
_____

DATE	GOAL PROGRESS REPORT
Current Date:	Goal:
1-Week evaluation	
2-Week evaluation	
3-Week evaluation	
4-Week evaluation	

DATE	GOAL PROGRESS REPORT
Current Date:	Goal:
1-Week evaluation	
2-Week evaluation	
3-Week evaluation	
4-Week evaluation	

DATE	GOAL PROGRESS REPORT
Current Date:	Goal:
1-Week evaluation	
2-Week evaluation	
3-Week evaluation	
4-Week evaluation	

Chapter **2** **Interpersonal Dynamics and Communications**

Problem-Solving Models

Use these sample stories to complete the problem-solving model in the space provided.

Problem 1: You receive your first test back in chemistry class. The grade is a D. You had taken notes during the class lectures, skimmed the chapter, and looked over your notes the night before the test. You had done most of the homework assignments and earned a C grade on them. You know that a grade of D in chemistry could prevent you from going on to an advanced program or college. You want to improve your grade.

Step 1: Recognize that a problem exists. What is the problem?	
Step 2: Clarify the issue. List who is involved and where, when, and how the problem occurred. What other factors affect it?	
Step 3: Identify alternative methods for resolving the problem.	
Step 4: Choose the best method for resolving the problem and implement it. (You may use your imagination to finish the problem.)	
Step 5: Evaluate the results of the method chosen. (You may use your imagination to finish the problem.)	

Problem 2: Describe a problem that you face in your school, work, or home situations. Use the problem-solving method to develop a solution.

Step 1: Recognize that a problem exists. What is the problem?	
Step 2: Clarify the issue. List who is involved and where, when, and how the problem occurred. What other factors affect it?	
Step 3: Identify alternative methods for resolving the problem.	
Step 4: Choose the best method for resolving the problem and implement it. (You may use your imagination to finish the problem.)	
Step 5: Evaluate the results of the method chosen. (You may use your imagination to finish the problem.)	

Team Building and Leadership

The jigsaw lesson plan is a way to build teams and to develop leadership skills. Work in groups of four for this activity. Each person in the group is assigned one of the tasks. The group task is to develop a fictitious experiment that demonstrates the effectiveness of communication forms. For example, the experiment might compare the effectiveness of written to verbal communication of a message.

Group Member One creates an illustration of the experiment.

Group Member Two creates the procedure list for the experiment.

Group Member Three creates a set of fictitious data in an appropriate format, such as a graph or data chart.

Group Member Four creates a 5- to 10-point quiz that tests understanding of the experiment and interpretation of the results.

Present the experiment to the class or another group as directed by the teacher. Use Boxes 2-9 and 2-11 in the textbook to describe the role you played in the jigsaw. Did you show the qualities of an effective leader or a good team member? Write a paragraph describing your role in this activity.

_____

_____

_____

_____

_____

Chapter **2 Interpersonal Dynamics and Communications**

Observing Communication Behaviors

In January 2009, Nadya Suleman gave birth to octuplets as a result of in vitro fertilization. This event caused a great deal of controversy over the ethics of Dr. Kamarava, her fertility specialist. Ms. Suleman was at the time an unemployed, single mother of six (all of in vitro fertilization). The hospital cost is estimated to be $2 million.

Dr. Kamarava stated that the decision to implant the embryos was based on (1) his love of children, (2) not wanting to discard the embryos, (3) the informed consent, and (4) his high value for choice.

In March of 2009, fifteen Kaiser Permanente Bellflower Medical Center workers were fired for accessing Ms. Suleman's health records without permission. Eight others face disciplinary action.

This event provides several topics of ethical debate in health care. Choose one of the following ethical issues. Break into groups based on the issue chosen and talk about it for 15 minutes.

- Ms. Suleman chose to have octuplets, although she was already unable to independently care for her other children.
- Dr. Kamarava chose to implant the embryos and bring all to birth knowing Ms. Suleman's situation and the risk of disorders in multiple birth babies.
- The hospital workers looked at the medical record of Ms. Suleman without permission.

Review Box 2-12 in the textbook. Use the guidelines describing attitudes and behaviors that are barriers to effective communication to observe conversations in your daily life. Describe at least five examples of barriers you observed in your own communication or that of others.

1. _____

_____

2. _____

_____

3. _____

_____

4. _____

_____

5. _____

_____

Questions

1. Which of the barriers that you observed can be easily changed?

_____

_____

_____

2. Why do you think that people use barriers in their communication with others?

_____

_____

_____

Practicing Telephone Etiquette

Work with a partner for this activity. Play the role of the client, with your partner acting as the receptionist in the following situations. The "client" may add information to the situation if desired. The "receptionist" may ask for any additional information needed. Evaluate your telephone technique by having the "receptionist" repeat the information gathered after all of the scenarios have been completed.

Situation 1: Your daughter, age 2 years, has been running a fever of 102° F all night. The child has been crying, and you have had very little sleep. You want to make an appointment to see the doctor as soon as possible.

Situation 2: You are calling to try to find a new veterinarian for your dog. A friend gave you the name of a practitioner. You would like to know the price of the services, the number of veterinarians in the practice and how long they have been practicing, and the hours that service is available. The availability of emergency care also is important to you. If the information you receive is satisfactory, you will make an appointment to have your dog vaccinated.

Situation 3: You are calling to make an appointment with the dentist for an annual checkup. You have been experiencing some cold sensations by one of your right molars, which you think may be a problem. It is important that you do not miss school for the appointment.

Situation 4: You are working as an assistant on a hospital unit. Although answering the phone is not part of your job, you are the only one in the area when the phone rings. The caller is a doctor wanting to leave admission orders for a client.

Situation 5: Invent and convey a message to your partner.

Questions

1. Was any part of the meaning of your message lost in your communication?

_____

_____

_____

2. How can you improve your ability to communicate clearly?

_____

_____

_____

CRITICAL THINKING

Time Management

Use the following chart to record the time you usually spend each day on the listed activities of daily living. Convert these estimated times to weekly percentages, and complete Figure 2-1. Each week has 10,080 minutes.

ACTIVITY	TIME IN MINUTES
Sleeping	
Eating	
Dressing/undressing	
Exercising	
Reading/study	
School/work	
Leisure activity	
Shopping/errands	
Other:	
Other:	

Chapter **2** **Interpersonal Dynamics and Communications**

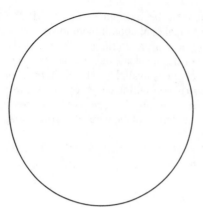

Figure 2-1

Questions

1. On which activity do you spend the most time?

_____

_____

_____

2. On which activity do you spend more time than you would prefer?

_____

_____

_____

3. On which activity do you spend less time than you would prefer?

_____

_____

_____

4. Can you make any changes in your daily activities that would allow you to spend more time on the activities you prefer?

_____

_____

_____

Ask the Right Question

The following are some situations in which the health care worker may not understand the thinking of the patient or co-worker. Formulate at least two questions to determine more information that would promote better health care.

1. You notice that the patient is not eating any of the food on the serving tray. When you ask why, the patient just shrugs and says he is not hungry. What are two questions you might ask?

_____

_____

2. Each day when you ask a patient if she would like to take a walk, she states that she is tired. What are two questions you might ask?

_____

_____

3. You notice that a co-worker does not go in the patient rooms or talk with any of the doctors when they visit the patients. What are two questions you might ask?

_____

_____

INTERNET ACTIVITIES

Game Development

Use the following web links to develop a game that teaches therapeutic humor as a method of stress reduction or a game that teaches listening skills. Describe the design of your game in the space provided.

Therapeutic Humor

Association for Applied Therapeutic Humor: http://aath.org/articles/index.html
Jest for the Health of It: http://www.jesthealth.com/resources.html

Game Design

_____

_____

_____

_____

_____

_____

Listening Skills

Lessons in Listening: http://7-12educators.about.com/gi/dynamic/offsite.htm?site=http://bbll.com/ch02.html
Active Listening: http://www.aligningaction.com/activeli.htm

Game Design

_____

_____

_____

_____

_____

_____

Online Career Survey

From the Arizona Department of Education Career Information website (http://www.azcis.intocareers.org/), choose the college link. Then choose the "Begin with occupation sort" under the "Earn a living at what you like to do" heading. Print (or open) the nine pages of the occupation sort worksheet. Follow the instructions to select the factors that are important to you.

Career Information website: http://www.azcis.intocareers.org/
Username: asucareer
Password: 4AZcis02

When finished, click the "Select Factors" link and follow the instructions to complete the occupation sort. List the 15 factors that are most important to you.

Chapter **2** **Interpersonal Dynamics and Communications**

Review two of the occupations that resulted from your survey. Write two paragraphs (minimum of seven sentences each). Each paragraph should describe one of the two occupations you chose from the list of occupations generated by your factors that are important in an occupation. Were any of the occupations in health care?

Most Important Factors

1. _____
2. _____
3. _____
4. _____
5. _____
6. _____
7. _____
8. _____
9. _____
10. _____
11. _____
12. _____
13. _____
14. _____
15. _____

Occupation 1

_____
_____
_____
_____
_____
_____
_____
_____

Occupation 2

_____
_____
_____
_____
_____
_____
_____
_____

3 ▍ Safety Practices

VAPID VOCABULARY

Complete the crossword puzzle using the Key Terms.

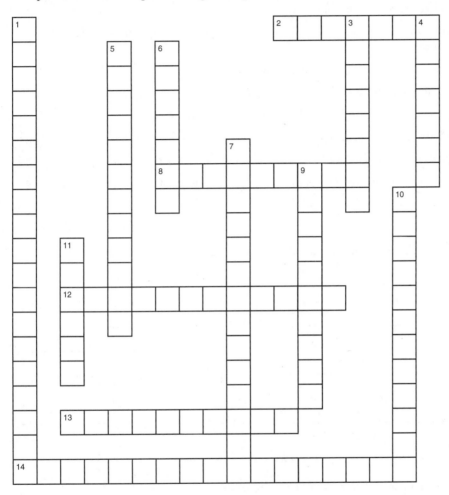

ACROSS

2 The methods used to prevent the spread of microorganisms
8 Unit that uses steam under pressure to sterilize materials
12 Soiled, made unclean, or infected with pathogens
13 Design of equipment for the workplace that maximizes productivity by reducing fatigue and discomfort
14 An infection located throughout the body (two words)

DOWN

1 CDC guidelines for infection control that are applied to all body fluids of all patients all of the time (two words)
3 Disease-causing microorganism
4 Free from living microorganisms
5 Substance that kills microorganisms except viruses and spores
6 An infectious disease of warm-blooded animals caused by a spore-forming bacterium
7 An infection limited to a small area of the body (two words)
9 Substance that deters the growth of microorganisms
10 CDC guidelines for infection control applied to patients with known or suspected infections (two words)
11 Organism that carries or transports a pathogen

ABBREVIATIONS

Match each of the following abbreviations with the phrase that best describes its meaning or function. Then write the phrase or name for each of the abbreviations in the spaces provided.

Abbreviation

1. _____ MRSA
2. _____ MSDS
3. _____ OBRA
4. _____ OSHA
5. _____ PASS
6. _____ POD
7. _____ PPE
8. _____ RACE
9. _____ UP
10. _____ VRE

Meaning or Function

a. Agency that regulates safety guidelines for a workplace

b. Antibiotic resistant enterococci infection

c. Antibiotic resistant *Staphylococcus* infection

d. Equipment, such as gloves, used by the health care worker to prevent the spread of pathogens

e. Law that requires training for nursing assistants

f. List of the contents, uses, and dangers of a chemical

g. Method used to clear a floor or building in case of fire

h. Method used to extinguish a fire

i. Methods used with all patients to prevent the spread of microorganisms

j. Place where medications or information is given to the public in an emergency

1. MRSA: _____

2. MSDS: _____

3. OBRA: _____

4. OSHA: _____

5. PASS: _____

6. POD: _____

7. PPE: _____

8. RACE: _____

9. UP: _____

10. VRE: _____

JUST THE FACTS

1. The six elements that must be present for infection to occur include pathogenic

   _ _ _ _ _ _ Ǫ _ _ _ _ _ _, a reservoir, a method of exit or escape, a means of

   _ _ _ _ Ǫ _ _ _ _ _ _ _, a method of entry, and a susceptible host.

2. Infection may be Ǫ _ _ _ _ _ _ _ _ _ _ _ or

   Ǫ _ _ _ _ _ _ _ _ _ _ _ _ _, local or general.

3. _ Ǫ _ _ _ _ _ Ǫ precautions are applied to all patients at all times and include all body fluids except perspiration.

4. The primary method of protection against infection is good _ _ Ǫ _ _ _ _ _ _ _ _ _ technique.

5. The most common method of transfer of pathogens causing serious illness in health care workers is contact with a

   _ _ Ǫ _ _ _ _ _ _ _ _ _ _ _ _ _ _ _ _ _ or _ _ _ _ _ instrument.

6. _ _ _ _ _ Ⓞ _ is the absence of disease-causing microorganisms.

7. OSHA establishes and enforces standards of Ⓞ _ _ _ _ _ for the workplace.

8. Ⓞ _ _ _ Ⓞ _ _ _ _ _ _ _ _ refers to the way the body is moved to prevent injury to oneself and to others.

9. The three elements that must be present for a fire to occur are Ⓞ _ _ _ _ _ _, _ _ Ⓞ _, and _ _ Ⓞ _.

10. Infectious and hazardous waste may be disposed of in the Ⓞ _ _ _ _ _ system or by Ⓞ _ _ _ _ _ _ _ _ _ _ _ _ _.

Use the circled letters to form the answer to this jumble. Clue: What are the isolation precautions based on specific types of illness called?

_ _ _ _ _ _ _ _ _ _ _ _ _ _ _ _·_ _ _ _ _

INVESTIGATIONS

Effectiveness of Handwashing

Read all directions before beginning this activity. Laboratory activities should be performed under the supervision of a qualified professional only.

Equipment and Supplies

Paper towels
Sink
Scrub brush (optional)
Soap
Ultraviolet light indicator
Ultraviolet light

Directions

1. Cover your hands with a spray or lotion that is visible under ultraviolet light only. Allow the solution to dry.
2. Following the skill list procedure found in the textbook, wash and dry your hands with water.
3. Observe your hands briefly under the ultraviolet light to determine whether any indicator was missed. Record your results.
4. Perform the activity again, using soap and water, to compare the effectiveness of this technique in removing the indicator.
5. Observe your hands briefly under the ultraviolet light to determine whether any indicator was missed. Record your results.
6. Perform the activity again, using water, soap, and a surgical scrub brush, to compare the effectiveness of this technique in removing the indicator.
7. Observe your hands briefly under the ultraviolet light to determine whether any indicator was missed. Record your results.
8. Continue washing your hands, if necessary, until all of the indicator have been removed.
9. Replace all equipment and supplies in the designated area.

MATERIALS USED	OBSERVATIONS
Water only	
Soap and water	
Soap, water, and brush	

Questions

1. Did you wash all areas of your hands equally well? If not, what areas did you miss?

_____

_____

_____

2. How did the effectiveness of washing with water alone compare to washing with soap and water?

_____

_____

_____

3. How did the effectiveness of washing with soap and water compare to washing with soap, water, and a surgical scrub brush?

_____

_____

_____

Comparing Hazards of Household Products

Prepare a list of the MSDS requirements for a common household item on a note card, excluding the name of the product. Compare and trade cards with classmates. Use the information to identify as many of the products as possible.

Questions

1. Which household items were you able to identify using the MSDS information?

_____

_____

2. Were any of the household items more or less dangerous than you expected?

_____

_____

3. Based on the information in the MSDS cards, will you use any of the products differently?

_____

_____

TEACHING PREPAREDNESS

Use a piece of white paper to create a pamphlet that illustrates the concepts of "R.A.C.E." and "PASS" in the school or health care facility setting. The pamphlet should be designed to educate the reader about these concepts. It should include emergency exits, equipment, and phone numbers that are appropriate to the facility chosen.

CRITICAL THINKING

Disease Detecting

The CDC has developed a curriculum for epidemiology. This set of modules allows students to use problem solving as disease detectives. Use the link to investigate an outbreak. Review each of the five student exercises and their answers.

http://www.cdc.gov/excite/classroom/outbreak/index.htm

After reviewing the CDC Disease Detective curriculum, use the following story to gather information about an outbreak of meningococcal infections at Penn State University in 2009. Use the information to answer question #3.

On February 12, 2009, Penn State University announced that two students had been hospitalized with meningococcal infections. One student died of the infection in 2007, but no cases had been reported since that time. Another student was hospitalized with the infection on February 13. It was determined that all three students had contact through their fraternity and sorority activities. More than 3000 students had similar contact with the hospitalized students. One of the three students was released from the hospital on February 16. Brown University sent an e-mail to its students that linked the outbreak to the Penn State University fencing team. No new cases of the infection have been reported.

Questions

1. What is an outbreak?

   _____

2. What are the steps of an outbreak investigation?

   _____

   _____

   _____

3. Use the disease detective curriculum to write a paragraph describing how to solve the Penn State meningococcal outbreak. Include:
   - Terms that need to be defined to understand the problem
   - Why the problem is important
   - What steps are needed to investigate the problem
   - The data that must be collected
   - A hypothesis about the cause of problem
   - What could be done to test the hypothesis

   _____

   _____

   _____

   _____

   _____

   _____

IDENTIFYING HAZARDS

Tour the health care facility, your home, or the school to create a list of safety hazards. Discuss the hazards identified by class members to determine their severity and any action needed to correct the problems noted.

CDC Case Study

The Bureau of Labor Statistics reported that 48% of all nonfatal injuries from workplace violence occurred in the health care industry. Most of the assaults occurred in nursing homes, hospitals, and places that provide residential care. The types of workers who have been assaulted include pharmacists, physicians, and nurses, as well as other workers.

The CDC has recognized risk factors for assault in the workplace. In 1989, OSHA established voluntary, generic safety and health program management guidelines for all employers.

Investigate the risk factors and guidelines established by the CDC and OSHA, using the web links that follow. Design a survey of questions based on the information gathered that could be used to rate the safety of the health care worker in a health care facility. Complete the survey for your school, and discuss safety issues in small groups as assigned by your instructor.

OSHA Report: Workplace Violence:

http://www.osha.gov/SLTC/workplaceviolence/

http://www.osha.gov/SLTC/etools/hospital/hazards/workplaceviolence/viol.html

OSHA Guidelines for Prevention:

http://www.osha.gov/SLTC/workplaceviolence/solutions.html

http://www.osha.gov/Publications/OSHA3148/osha3148.html

Questions

1. What are the risk factors of workplace violence?

_____

_____

_____

_____

_____

2. What guidelines were established by the CDC and OSHA regarding workplace violence?

_____

_____

_____

_____

_____

3. List five questions that might be included in a survey of a health care facility to rate its level of safety.

_____

_____

_____

_____

_____

_____

_____

4. Complete the workplace safety quiz from the following link. Record your score.

http://nonprofitrisk.org/tools/workplace-safety/nonprofit/wsp.htm

Score: _____

THE CHALLENGE OF THE PRIONS

Prions are the only known "organism" that can reproduce without nucleic acids. They are proteins that change the metabolism of a cell. An example of a disease caused by a prion is bovine spongiform encephalopathy (BSE), or "mad cow disease." An epidemic of BSE began in Great Britain in 1985. Variant Creutzfeldt-Jakob disease (vCJD) is a human disorder that appeared after the epidemic of mad cow disease (BSE) in Great Britain. It has been suggested that the victims of vCJD acquired the disease from eating contaminated beef. However, CJD is also an inherited disease in 10% to 15% of cases, and most of the cases are sporadic CJD (sCJD) with no known cause. Graft and corneal transplant recipients have acquired CJD from a person who inherited the disease.

One of the challenges in health care that has resulted from the appearance of prion-caused diseases is their resistance to sterilization. Use the Internet links that follow to research this condition, and write an essay describing your findings.

Some concepts to include in the essay are:
- Examples of other diseases caused by prions
- The number of cases that have occurred
- Examples of transmission to and from humans to other animals
- Signs and symptoms of prion infection
- Isolation and sterilization procedures used by health care workers
  Creutzfeldt-Jakob Disease Foundation: http://www.cjdfoundation.org/
  CDC: http://www.cdc.gov/ncidod/dvrd/prions/

Essay

4 Legal and Ethical Principles

VAPID VOCABULARY

Complete the crossword puzzle using the Key Terms.

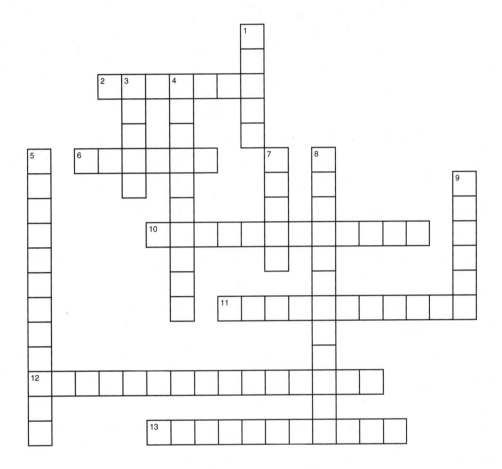

ACROSS

2 Verbally communicating something untruthful and harmful about another person
6 Legally responsible
10 Use of telecommunications technology to provide, improve, or make health care services faster
11 Study of information processing, computer science
12 Agreement to surgical or medical treatment with knowledge of facts and risks involved (two words)
13 Failure of professtional skill or learning that results in injury, loss, or damage

DOWN

1 Relating to principles of right and wrong
3 Deriving authority from or founded on law
4 Failure to execute the care that a reasonable (prudent) person exercises
5 Private or secret
7 Communicating something untruthful and harmful about another person in writing
8 Understanding the science or philosophy of law
9 Dealing with what is good or bad, determining moral duty and obligation

ABBREVIATIONS

Match each of the following abbreviations with the phrase that best describes its meaning or function. Then write the phrase or name for each of the abbreviations in the spaces provided.

Abbreviation

1. _____ AHA
2. _____ DNR
3. _____ DRG
4. _____ EMR
5. _____ HHS
6. _____ HIPAA
7. _____ JCAHO
8. _____ NPA
9. _____ OCR
10. _____ PHI

Meaning or Function

a. Agency that adopted the Patient's Bill of Rights

b. Agency that approves health care organizations

c. Any individual identifiable information

d. Digital record of patient care

e. Government agency responsible for protecting health of Americans and providing essential services

f. Government agency that enforces HIPAA rules

g. Law that determines what tasks nurses can do

h. Medical order to not revive a patient in case of cardiac arrest

i. Privacy rules

j. System to classify hospital cases to assess expected cost

1. AHA: _____

2. DNR: _____

3. DRG: _____

4. EMR: _____

5. HHS: _____

6. HIPAA: _____

7. JCAHO: _____

8. NPA: _____

9. OCR: _____

10. PHI: _____

JUST THE FACTS

1. Ethical practices include respect for the ⊖ _ _ _ _ _ ⊖ _, _ _ ⊖ _ _ _, and _ _ _ ⊖ _ _ differences of clients and other workers.

2. Morals are based on the experience, religion, and philosophy of the _ ⊖ _ _ ⊖ _ _ _ _ _ and _ _ _ _ _ _ ⊖.

3. Workers in every health care occupation are legally ⊖ _ _ _ _ ⊖ _ _ _ _ _ (liable) for their behavior and the care given.

4. The duties that may be performed by the health care worker depend on the level of ⊖ _ _ _ _ _ _ _ and _ _ _ _ ⊖ _ _ _ _ of the worker.

5. It is _ _ ⊖ _ _ _ _ _ _ _ _ to perform skills for which the health care worker does not have education and training.

6. In 1996, a _ _ _ _ _ _ _ _ law was passed to protect individually identifiable health information using _ _ _ _ _ _ _ _ _ _ _ technology.

7. The Privacy of Individually _ Ⓞ _ _ _ _ Ⓞ _ _ _ _ _ Health Information standards protect _ _ _ Ⓞ _ _ _ records and Ⓞ _ _ _ _ _ _ _ _ _ _ _ Ⓞ _ _ _ information.

8. Two types of advance directives are the _ Ⓞ _ _ _ _ _ Ⓞ _ _ and _ _ _ Ⓞ _ of _ _ _ Ⓞ _ _ _ Ⓞ.

9. _ _ _ _ Ⓞ _ _ _ in health care must be precise, clear, and concise.

10. The client's health information is communicated using _ _ _ _ _ _ Ⓞ _ _ and _ _ _ _ _ Ⓞ _ _ _.

Use the circled letters to form the answer to this jumble. Clue: What do the rights of any citizen of the United States include?

_ _ _ _ _ _ _   _ _ _   _

CONCEPT APPLICATIONS

In the News
Use a newspaper, magazine, or Internet article that describes a current legal or ethical case relating to the health care industry. Complete the information regarding the article in the designated spaces.

1. Title of article

_____

2. Name of publication

_____

3. Date of publication

_____

4. What is the legal breach or issue in dispute in the case described in the article?

_____

_____

_____

5. Summarize the plaintiff's point of view in the case.

_____

_____

_____

6. Summarize the defendant's point of view in the case.

_____

_____

_____

7. Predict the outcome of this legal dispute based on the information provided in the article.

_____

_____

_____

Classifying Conduct

In the following situations, identify whether a legal or ethical breach of conduct is described. Circle the word that corresponds to your choice. If the breach is a legal consideration, explain which crime has occurred. Use the table of Legal and Ethical Terminology in the textbook for reference.

1. A client in the hospital is angry about her care. She rings her bell 10 or more times an hour. You decide that she is just seeking attention, and you ignore the bell.

   Legal or Ethical Explanation:

   _____

   _____

   _____

2. You are helping a nurse who is changing a dressing on a client's wound, and you drop the sterile dressing on the floor. You know that no one saw the dressing drop, and you replace it on the sterile tray to save time and avoid getting into trouble.

   Legal or Ethical Explanation:

   _____

   _____

   _____

3. On arriving home, you find that you have accidentally taken a pen and a roll of tape from work. You decide they are not worth returning and place them in your drawer for use at home.

   Legal or Ethical Explanation:

   _____

   _____

   _____

4. You tell your best friend that, in your role as a student health care worker, you saw a student from your school admitted to the hospital because of an overdose. You name the student who was admitted, and your friend promises not to tell anyone else about it. Your friend does not tell anyone.

   Legal or Ethical Explanation:

   _____

   _____

   _____

5. You observe a family in the emergency department after an accident in which one of the children was injured. The family acts very dramatically by crying and clinging to the hospital staff. You mimic that family's reaction for your friends during the football game that evening.

   Legal or Ethical Explanation:

   _____

   _____

   _____

Understanding HIPAA

Obtain a copy of the HIPAA regulations or a release form used by a health care facility. Design a pamphlet to teach the content of the law to someone. Use the pamphlet to explain the law to a student in the class as directed by the instructor.

Planning Legal and Ethical Strategies

Read the following situations, which could create legal and ethical dilemmas in the health care setting. Describe how you would handle the situation, and justify your answer in the space provided. Discuss your choices with a partner or the group as directed by your instructor.

Situation 1: You observe that one of your co-workers routinely takes items such as pens and paper clips home in her pockets. She comments to you that she uses them for her kids and feels that, with her salary, it is the least the facility can contribute to her kids' education.

1. How would you handle this situation?

_____

_____

2. What is your reason for your choice of action?

_____

_____

Situation 2: One of the clients, Mrs. Standwell, is often confused and has difficulty with motor functions, such as walking. The family has forbidden the institution to restrain her. You find her after she has fallen and bruised her leg.

1. How would you handle this situation?

_____

_____

2. What is your reason for your choice of action?

_____

_____

Situation 3: One client in a double room has difficulty hearing and keeps the television volume high. The other roommate complains that the noise gives him a headache.

1. How would you handle this situation?

_____

_____

2. What is your reason for your choice of action?

_____

_____

Situation 4: After the morning break, you smell alcohol on the breath of one of your co-workers.

1. How would you handle this situation?

_____

_____

2. What is your reason for your choice of action?

_____

_____

Situation 5: One of the clients tells you that no one came into the room or checked on her throughout the night. She states that even her sleeping pill was omitted.

1. How would you handle this situation?

_____

_____

2. What is your reason for your choice of action?

_____

_____

Situation 6: Mrs. Cheats asks you to bring her some salt for her breakfast eggs. She does not have a diet card with her tray, and she has no apparent disorder except the use of oxygen by nasal prongs. You bring her the salt. After she has poured salt on the eggs, she laughs and states, "Ha, I'm not supposed to have salt because of my high blood pressure. Boy, are you in trouble."

1. How would you handle this situation?

_____

_____

2. What is your reason for your choice of action?

_____

_____

Situation 7: As you are walking by Mrs. Gripe's room, you hear one of your co-workers shout, "Shut up and move it or you'll be sorry."

1. How would you handle this situation?

_____

_____

2. What is your reason for your choice of action?

_____

_____

Situation 8: One of your clients is confused and frequently wanders out of his room, stating that he is "going home now." You are short of help and have concerns that he will leave the building.

1. How would you handle this situation?

_____

_____

2. What is your reason for your choice of action?

_____

_____

Situation 9: One of your clients is a jeweler, and he gives you a ring that he made as a token of appreciation for the care you have given him.

1. How would you handle this situation?

_____

_____

2. What is your reason for your choice of action?

_____

_____

Situation 10: You notice that one of your co-workers seems to get daily care and vital signs done early every day. A little more observation makes you aware that the person is not changing sheets daily and does not really take the vital signs of many of the clients.

1. How would you handle this situation?

_____

_____

2. What is your reason for your choice of action?

_____

_____

You Be the Judge

Verdict 1

In July 1991, a surgeon at the Osteopathic Medical Center in Fort Worth, Texas, removed the cancerous right lung of Benjamin H. Jones, Jr., age 59 years. Unfortunately, an altered test report and prodding by a colleague during the operation led to the removal of the wrong lung.

After the pathology examination confirmed that a healthy lung had been removed in error, no one informed Mr. Jones as to what had happened. Court records demonstrated that a top official at the hospital was informed of the discrepancy between the cancer screening and surgery results. The official stated that he relied on the doctors to inform Mr. Jones of the mix-up.

Two medical experts swore that Mr. Jones would have had a 60% chance of survival, even with the cancerous lung only, if he had received radiation therapy. At the time of the surgery, the cancer had not spread past the tumor. Mr. Jones died in February, 1992.

The Jones family settled out of court for $5.5 million with seven defendants in a wrongful death suit. Along with 20 other defendants, the hospital declined to settle.

Mr. Jones had begun smoking in his teens and had quit after suffering a heart attack about 7 years before the surgery.

Questions

1. What was the breach of law in this case?

_____

_____

2. In your opinion, who was legally responsible for Mr. Jones's death and why?

_____

_____

3. What safeguards might be used to prevent this type of mistreatment in a hospital?

_____

_____

4. In your opinion, was the settlement in this case fair?

_____

_____

Verdict 2

In September 1993, Fairfax Hospital in Virginia began to appeal a prior federal court's ruling that it must continue to provide life-sustaining treatment for an anencephalic baby born 11 months earlier. The baby was born with a brain stem that supported respiration and heart activity, but the infant had no cortex. Without a cortex, the baby never had consciousness, sensation, or the ability to think.

After birth, the baby was periodically taken from the nursing home in which he lived to the hospital for treatment of respiratory crisis and to be placed on a respirator. The hospital wanted to decline care for the baby. The American Academy of Pediatrics filed a brief supporting the hospital's position that life-sustaining treatment of this baby was inappropriate.

The mother insisted that the baby be kept alive, contrary to the recommendations of the doctors and medical ethics board of the hospital. In fact, the abnormality had been detected before birth, and the mother had declined abortion. The baby's father, who had never been married to the mother, supported the hospital's position.

The court decided that refusing treatment violated the Americans with Disabilities Act and the mother's Fourteenth Amendment right to "bring up children." The cost of the baby's care, approximately $1,500 a day, was provided by the mother's health maintenance organization.

Questions

1. Most cases involving treatment of severely damaged children raise the question of terminating life instead of prolonging life, as in this case. What is the central issue in both circumstances?

_____

_____

2. Why do you think the judge gave the most authority to the mother in determining care for this baby?

_____

_____

3. Which of the facts regarding this case do you feel are most important to making a decision about it?

_____

_____

Scope of Practice

Use the Internet to research the scope of practice of a nurse assistant, registered nurse, or other health care practitioner. Discuss the scope of practice of the chosen occupation with class members as directed by your instructor.

Abandonment

After hurricane Katrina passed through New Orleans, 34 residents of St. Rita's Nursing Home were found dead in the floodwaters. The owners were charged with negligent homicide. They had been offered buses to evacuate the residents but turned the offer down. *The New York Times* reported that at least 91 patients in hospitals and 62 in nursing homes were not evacuated until 5 days after the storm.

At the Memorial Medical Center, 45 patients were found dead after the storm. Health care workers from the center said that a doctor and two nurses injected some of the patients with lethal drugs. A year later, the doctor, Anna Pou, and two nurses were arrested for their acts, but the jury declined to indict them for second-degree murder. Dr. Pou has since helped write and pass laws in Louisiana that offer immunity from civil lawsuits for health care professionals for their work during a disaster.

Using the Internet, investigate what the requirements of "patient abandonment" include and one of the following issues. Write an essay that describes what your action would be in a similar situation.

Key Terms: nurse, abandonment, patient, Katrina

Issue #1: Dr. Pou says the standards of medical care should be different in emergencies such as hurricanes, pandemic outbreaks, and military action. For example, she states that informed consent is not possible, and that the sickest, most injured and those with DNR orders should be evacuated last.

Issue #2: Some health care workers did not report to work during the Katrina disaster. Instead, they took care of or left with their families.

Issue #3: Management of a health care facility that is short staffed may accuse a nurse or health care worker with patient abandonment. A nurse might be asked to work mandatory overtime or in an area for which the nurse is not trained or qualified.

Issue #4: Johns Hopkins Bloomberg School of Public Health conducted a study in 2009 that indicated that one in six public health care workers would not help in a pandemic flu emergency. A similar study they had conducted in 2005 indicated that 40% would not report to work.

Essay

_____

5 | Culture and Health Care

Complete the crossword puzzle using the Key Terms.

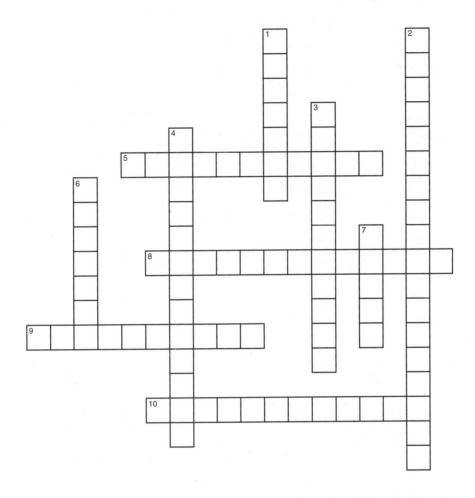

ACROSS

5 Society or group with a female as head of the family or tribal line
8 The process of learning cultural behaviors from one group or person
9 Simplified image used to characterize or describe a group
10 The merging of cultural traits from different cultural groups

DOWN

1 The act of belonging to a designated group
2 The ability to meet the health care needs of patients while meeting and adhering to their cultural values, beliefs, and practices (two words)
3 A branch of anthropology that studies and records various human culture
4 The belief that one's own culture is superior to another
6 Expressing or exciting emotion
7 Free from passion, without complaint

ABBREVIATIONS

Match each of the following abbreviations with the phrase that best describes its meaning or function. Then write the phrase or name for each of the abbreviations in the spaces provided.

Abbreviation	Meaning or Function
1. _____ CDC	a. Federal agency that determines safety of medications
2. _____ FDA	b. Federal agency that investigates illnesses
3. _____ H1N1	c. Federal agency that oversees American health
4. _____ HHS	d. HHS agency that manages health care for Native Americans
5. _____ IHS	e. Nonprofit organization that works to prevent medication error
6. _____ ISMP	f. Person that is not fluent in English
7. _____ LEP	g. Type of influenza

1. CDC: _____

2. FDA: _____

3. H1N1: _____

4. HHS: _____

5. IHS: _____

6. ISMP: _____

7. LEP: _____

JUST THE FACTS

1. _ _ _ _ _ _ refers to the norms and practices of a particular group that are learned, _ _ _ _ _ _, and transcended through generations.

2. It is important to be _ _ _ _ _ of those beliefs and attitudes and be willing to accept patients' beliefs in order to care for them.

3. What may be considered _ _ _ _ _ _ _ _ _ _ to one group is healthy and normal for another.

4. Always ask _ _ _ _ _ _ _ _ _ _ first before _ _ _ _ _ _ _ _ _ any patient, regardless of cultural differences.

5. Before entering any patient's room, all health care team members should _ _ _ _ _ _ _ _ their arrival and wait a few moments before entering.

6. Patients often ask for and want visits from their _ _ _ _ _ _ _ _ _ leaders while hospitalized.

7. Some cultures welcome _ _ _ _ _ and see it as "advancing to the next _ _ _ _ _ _."

8. Some cultures view health care professionals as _ _ _ _ _ _ _ _ _ and thus may avoid any form of _ _ _ _ _ _ _ _ _ _ _ _ or discussion.

9. Stereotyping can lead to _ _ _ _ _ _ _ _ _, which leads to discrimination.

10. It is important to recognize that other cultures are not as Ⓞ _ _ _ - _ Ⓞ _ _ _ _ _ — _ _ as Americans.

Use the circled letters to form the answer to this jumble. Clue: What are two important factors in health care that can be lost if cultural differences are ignored?

_ _ _ _ _   _ _ _   _ _ _ _ _ _

CONCEPT APPLICATIONS

Self-Evaluation

Complete the following chart of cultural values. There are no "right" or "wrong" answers to this survey. Answer the questions based on your results.

YES	NO	CULTURAL BEHAVIOR SURVEY
		I am always on time.
		I am not embarrassed when health care workers see me without my clothes.
		I attend a religious institution regularly.
		I bathe every day.
		I believe everyone should speak English.
		I believe managing pain is largely a matter of willpower.
		I believe men should be the head of the household.
		I believe my religion is the way to reach eternal life.
		I believe people should not touch another person's infant without being asked first.
		I believe poor grammar is a sign of ignorance.
		I believe prayer is essential to healing.
		I believe suicide is an unforgivable sin.
		I do not eat certain foods because of my religion.
		I do not eat meat.
		I do not like people to touch me.
		I do not like to undress in front of anyone.
		I do not speak English in my home.
		I eat any type of food and have no cultural requirements.
		I feel uncomfortable when I have to sit next to someone of the opposite sex whom I do not know.
		I feel uncomfortable when I sit next to someone of a different race whom I do not know.
		I follow a diet determined by my religion.
		I see a doctor when necessary and follow directions given to me.
		I think death is the end of existence.
		I think men or women who wear scanty clothes have bad moral values.
		I think overweight people are lazy.
		I think people should not be allowed to have same-sex marriages.
		I think people who change their gender are sick.
		I think people who have pierced their body have bad moral values.
		I think prayer and religion should not be practiced in public.
		I touch people when I talk with them.
		I use my hands and gestures to communicate.
		I use some words and phrases that are specific to my ethnic or religious beliefs or group.
		I wear clothes that are conservative.

Questions

1. Describe how you were surprised by any of the answers you gave in the survey

_____

_____

2. Explain from what or how your beliefs were formed.

_____

_____

3. Describe how one of your beliefs has affected the way you have treated another person.

_____

_____

INVESTIGATIONS

Observing Cultural Behaviors

Write a paragraph that describes one cultural or religious behavior that you have observed in another person but did not understand. Use the Internet to research the origin of the behavior. Discuss the results of your research with members of the class as directed by the instructor.

_____

_____

_____

_____

_____

_____

CRITICAL THINKING

Pair and Share

Round One

Form pairs in groups of eight. Spend five minutes each discussing each of the following topics with that person. Form a new pair with a different individual to discuss the second topic for five minutes. Form a new pair to discuss the third and fourth topics.

Pair #1: Discuss your cultural background and how it was reflected in the cultural survey.
Pair #2: Discuss the traits of your culture of which you are proud.
Pair #3: Describe someone of your culture (not family) that has been a good role model for you and others.
Pair #4: Describe a time when you felt uncomfortable because of your cultural background.

Round Two

Imagine you are a member of a different cultural group. Repeat the pair/share process answering from the perspective of a member of that cultural group.

Questions

1. Did you feel that you knew enough about the imagined culture to discuss the topic well? Where did you get your information?

_____

_____

2. What characteristics did you use to choose a good role model for this activity?

_____

_____

Cultural Understanding

Some politicians and religious leaders believe that some religious and cultural differences cannot be resolved by any method except destruction of the people who do not share the same religion or culture. Write a paragraph that describes your belief regarding this issue. Discuss your paragraph with class members as directed by your instructor.

_____

_____

_____

_____

_____

_____

_____

INTERNET ACTIVITIES

Community Research

Use the following links and a search of the Internet to determine the composition of the local community. Answer the questions based on your research.

U.S. Census Bureau Data Profiles: http://quickfacts.census.gov/qfd/index.html

State Facts for Students: http://www.census.gov/schools/facts/

City data: http://www.city-data.com/

Questions

1. What is the proportion of cultural groups in your area?

_____

_____

_____

2. Compare the demographical (cultural, ethnic, or religious) composition of the class to your community, city, or state statistics.

_____

_____

_____

CLAS Standards

The Office of Minority Health (OMH) developed 14 standards for culturally appropriate services for health care organizations. They are called the _National Standards for Culturally and Linguistically Appropriate Services (CLAS)_. Use the following links to review the standards, and restate each of the themes in your own words.

http://minorityhealth.hhs.gov/templates/browse.aspx?lvl=2&lvlID=15

https://www.thinkculturalhealth.org/Documents/CLAS_Standards.pdf

THEME	DESCRIPTION
Culturally Competent Care (Standards 1-3)	
Language Access Services (Standards 4-7)	
Organizational Supports for Cultural Competence (Standards 8-14)	

Questions

1. Describe how each of the themes can be applied to the individual health care worker as well as to the organization.

_____

_____

_____

2. Describe how your experiences with health care have met or missed the standards set by CLAS.

_____

_____

_____

Improving Cultural Competence

In a Public Health Reports article of July–August 2003, the author suggests there are three aspects or parts of health care that lead to sociocultural barriers in health care. These include organizational barriers, structural barriers, and clinical barriers. For example, the article reports that, although Latinos, African Americans, and Native Americans make up 28% of the population, only 2% of people with senior leadership roles in health care are non-white. That is an organizational barrier. Structural barriers include things such as a lack of interpreter services and long wait times for service. Clinical barriers have to do with the health care worker's interaction with the patient.

Use the Internet to investigate the programs that have been developed to improve cultural competence in health care. Write an essay that describes the program, the sociocultural barrier it addresses, and information about its success.

Office of Minority Health: http://minorityhealth.hhs.gov/templates/browse.aspx?lvl=1&lvlID=3

Essay

_____

_____

_____

_____

_____

_____

_____

_____

_____

_____

_____

_____

_____

_____

_____

_____

_____

_____

_____

_____

VAPID VOCABULARY

Complete the crossword puzzle using the Key Terms.

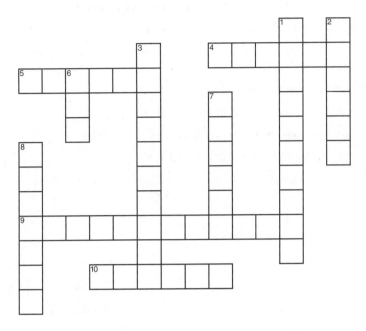

ACROSS

4 Discuss a question
5 Proposal for action
9 A structure through which individuals cooperate systematically to conduct business
10 List of things to be done or considered, program of work

DOWN

1 To disturb persistently, torment, bother, or persecute
2 Brief summary of professional and work experience
3 Energy or aptitude for action, enterprise
6 Contribution to the support of government, fee, or dues of an organization to pay its expenses
7 Summary of projected income and expenses
8 To suspend a session to another time or permanently

ABBREVIATIONS

Match each of the following abbreviations with the phrase that best describes its meaning or function. Then write the phrase or name for each of the abbreviations in the spaces provided.

Abbreviation

Meaning or Function

1. _____ CERT

   a. FEMA training program to learn about emergency preparedness and disaster response

2. _____ CMS-1500

   b. Medicare insurance form

3. _____ CPR

   c. Model used to answer behavior interview questions that include evaluation

4. _____ FICA

   d. Model used to answer behavior interview questions that include the task

5. _____ HOSA

   e. Model used to answer behavior interview questions that include the problem, action, and result

6. _____ MRC

   f. Rescue procedure for someone with cardiac arrest

7. _____ PAR

   g. Student organization that includes health and trade occupations

8. _____ SHARE

   h. Student-led organization, including leadership and skill training in health careers only

9. _____ SkillsUSA

   i. Taxes paid by employer and employee to fund Social Security

10. _____ STAR

   j. Volunteer program organized to respond to natural disasters and emergencies

1. CERT: _____

2. CMS-1500: _____

3. CPR: _____

4. FICA: _____

5. HOSA: _____

6. MRC: _____

7. PAR: _____

8. SHARE: _____

9. SkillsUSA: _____

10. STAR: _____

JUST THE FACTS

1. In an organization, a group of individuals join together to reach a goal by ◯ _ _ _ _ _ _ _ _ _ _ _ and division of ◯ _ _ _ _ among themselves.

2. Work is a means of self-fulfillment and a method to earn a _ _ ◯ _ _ _ and establish economic _ _ _ _ _ _ _ _ _.

3. Benefits of membership in a student organization include the exchange of information with others who have similar interests, an opportunity to _ ◯ _ _ _ _ _ _ _ ◯ _ _ _ through competition, and a way to develop _ _ _ _ _ _ _ _ _ _ ability.

4. One of the elements of an effective group is a clear understanding of its ◯ _ _ _ _ _ _ _ and _ _ ◯ _ _.

5. Parliamentary procedure maintains a sense of order during meetings and ensures that all

   _ _ _ _ _ _ _ have a chance to participate _ _ _ _ _ _ _.

6. Employers use the _ _ _ _ Ⓞ _ _ _ _ _ _, résumé, and

   _ _ _ _ _ _ _ _ _ _ to determine who is the best applicant.

7. Many prospective employees do not recognize that the first interview occurs when the

   _ Ⓞ _ _ _ _ _ _ _ _ _ _ is obtained from the

   _ _ _ _ _ Ⓞ _ _ _ _ _ _.

8. To determine whether an employment opportunity will provide for an employee's needs, a

   _ _ _ _ Ⓞ _ _ _ _ _ _ _ _ _ may be used to determine whether these financial
   goals can be met.

9. Deductions that may be taken from the paycheck before the employee receives it include _ _ _ _ _,

   social security, and _ Ⓞ _ _ _ _ _ _ _ costs.

10. Most people who lose a job after being hired do so because of _ _ _ _ _ _ _ Ⓞ rather than

    Ⓞ _ _ _ _ _ _ to do the job.

   Use the circled letters to form the answer to this jumble. Clue: What is the first sample of the quality of an employee's work?

   _ _ _ _ _ _ _ _ _ _ _ _ _ _ _ _.

CONCEPT APPLICATIONS

Balancing a Checkbook

Use the information provided in Figure 6-1 to balance the checkbook register.

CHECK NO.	DATE	CHECK ISSUED TO OR DEPOSIT RECEIVED FROM	AMOUNT OF CHECK	X	AMOUNT OF DEPOSIT	BALANCE 1058.36
ATM	1/1	Cash-groceries	$100.00	X		$958.36
ATM	1/1	Paycheck		X	$1,523.46	
104	1/5	Telephone	$24.98	X		
105	1/5	Electric	$104.36	X		
106	1/5	Rent	$1,023.00	X		
107	1/10	Car Insurance-6 months	$525.00			
ATM	1/15	Paycheck			$1,523.46	
108	1/19	Cable-TV	$49.63			
109	1/19	Car payment	$105.68			
ATM	1/19	Cash-groceries	$100.00			

Figure 6-1

Questions

1. What is the balance of this checkbook on 1/19?

   _____

2. Which is the largest expense incurred this month, as indicated by the check register?

   _____

3. Which of the expenses is a luxury (i.e., not a necessity)?

_____

4. Is the individual with this checkbook living "within his or her means"? Justify your response using examples from the register.

_____

_____

_____

Creating a Personal Financial Statement

Use Figure 6-2 to create a personal financial statement.

PERSONAL FINANCIAL STATEMENT

Owned:

Cash	$ _____
Securities (stocks, bonds, CDs)	$ _____ *
Real estate	$ _____ *
Automobile	$ _____ *
Furniture	$ _____ *
Receivables (money owed to you)	$ _____
Other	$ _____

Total Owned: $ _____

Owed:

Household bills unpaid	$ _____
Installment payments:	
Automobile	$ _____
Appliances	$ _____
Loans	$ _____
Other	$ _____
Real estate payments	$ _____
Insurance:	
Automobile	$ _____
Personal property	$ _____
Health	$ _____
Other	$ _____
Taxes	$ _____
Other debts	$ _____

Total Owed: $ _____

Total Owned Minus Total Owed Equals Total Worth = $ _____

*Value should be determined by the amount that could be obtained from a quick sale.

Figure 6-2

Questions

1. If your total worth is more than your total debt, what would be a good way to invest the excess income?

_____

_____

_____

2. If your total worth is less than your total debt, what would be a source of additional money or an expense that could be cut?

_____

_____

_____

Planning a Budget

Use Figure 6-3 to create a personal budget. Allow at least 6% for savings.

Questions

1. List three expenses that are discretionary but necessary.

_____

_____

_____

2. Explain why it is more (or less) expensive to eat in a restaurant than at home.

_____

_____

_____

3. What are two ways in which you could reduce your personal expenses without giving up discretionary expenditures that are important to you?

_____

_____

_____

Regular or Fixed Monthly Payments*

Mortgage or rent	$ _____
Automobile payment	$ _____
Automobile insurance	$ _____
Appliance	$ _____
Loan	$ _____
Health insurance	$ _____
Personal property insurance	$ _____
Telephone	$ _____
Utilities (gas or electric)	$ _____
Water	$ _____
Other non-emergency expenses	$ _____

Discretionary or Variable Payments

Clothing, laundry, cleaning	$ _____
Medicine	$ _____
Doctor and dentist	$ _____
Education	$ _____
Dues	$ _____
Gifts and donations	$ _____
Travel	$ _____
Subscriptions	$ _____
Automobile maintenance and gas	$ _____
Spending money and entertainment	$ _____

Food Expenses

Food—at home	$ _____
Food—away from home	$ _____

Taxes

Federal and state income tax	$ _____
Property	$ _____
Other taxes	$ _____

Other

Other	$ _____

TOTAL MONTHLY PAYMENTS $ _____

SAMPLE RECOMMENDED BUDGET EXPENDITURES

Shelter (rent or mortgage)	20%
Food	25%
Clothing	12%
Transportation	12%
Medical and dental	6%
Dues and charities	9%
Education and entertainment	10%
Savings	6%*

---

* Financial advisers recommend that savings should cover expenses for at least 3 months.

Figure 6-3

Chapter **6** **Employability Skills**

Planning for Business Meetings

Use Figure 6-4 to complete an agenda for conducting a meeting of your student organization. Conduct a meeting of the organization using the agenda. Use Figure 6-5 to record the secretary's minutes and Figure 6-6 to create a treasurer's report.

AGENDA

BUSINESS ITEM	PERSON RESPONSIBLE
I. Call to Order	Presiding officer: _____
II. Invocation (optional)	Designated officer: _____
III. Pledge of Allegiance (optional)	Presiding officer: _____
IV. Roll Call/Establish Quorum	Secretary: _____
V. Minutes of Previous Meeting	Secretary: _____
VI. Treasurer's Report	Treasurer: _____
VII. Officers' Reports	Vice president: _____
	Others: _____
VIII. Committee Reports A. Standing Committees	Committee chairs: _____
1. Fund Raising	Committee chair: _____
2. Membership	Committee chair: _____
3. Social B. Special	Committee chair: _____
1. Health Fair	Committee chair: _____
2. Field Trip	Committee chair: _____
IX. Unfinished Business	Presiding officer: _____
X. New Business	Presiding officer: _____
XI. Program (optional)	Guest speaker: _____
XII. Announcements	Presiding officer: _____
XIII. Adjournment	Presiding officer: _____

Figure 6-4

```
Minutes of the Meeting of _____

_____ (date)

   The meeting was called to order at _____ (time). The minutes were

approved _____ (with/without) changes. The treasurer's report was

read and filed for audit.

   The _____(committee or individual) moved to _____

_____ (motion). Discussion was held. The motion

(carried/failed to carry) with a majority vote.

   The meeting was adjourned at _____ (time).

Respectfully submitted,

_____ (secretary)
```

Figure 6-5

Treasurer's Report

From _____(Date) to   (Date) _____
Income
   Membership dues: _____ $ _____
   Fees:_____ $ _____
   Interest:_____ $ _____
   Sales projects: _____ $ _____
                                       $ _____
   _____ $ _____
   Other: _____ $ _____
   _____ $ _____
   _____ $ _____
   Total income: _____ $ _____
Expenditures:
   Membership dues: _____ $ _____
   Fees:_____ $ _____
   Taxes:_____ $ _____
   Sales projects: _____ $ _____

   _____ $ _____
   _____ $ _____
   Other: _____ $ _____
   _____ $ _____
   _____ $ _____
   Total expenditures:_____ $ _____
   Beginning balance _____ $ _____
   Total income: _____ $ _____
   Sum: _____ $ _____
   Total expenditures: _____ $ _____
   Ending balance: _____ $ _____

Respectfully Submitted,

_____(Treasurer)

Figure 6-6

Preparing a Résumé

Use Figure 6-7 to complete a draft of a personal data sheet or résumé. Proofread and complete it according to your teacher's instructions.

Personal Data Sheet

Complete the following personal date sheet to assist you in filling out job applications. Employment and educational information should be presented with most current information first. References should be presented in alphabetical order.

_____

(Your Complete Name)

_____

(Address)

_____

(City, State, Zip Code)

_____

(Telephone Number)

Career Objective:

_____

Education

_____

(School, City, State, Years Attended)

_____

(School, City, State, Years Attended)

_____

(School, City, State, Years Attended)

Work Experience

_____

(Place of Employment, Dates Employed)

_____

(Place of Employment, Dates Employed)

Job-Related Skills and Training

_____ _____

_____ _____

_____ _____

_____ _____

Honors and Organizations

_____ _____

_____ _____

_____ _____

_____ _____

Personal Interests and Hobbies

_____ _____

_____ _____

_____ _____

_____ _____

References

_____

(Name, Occupation, Address, City, State, Zip Code, Telephone)

_____

(Name, Occupation, Address, City, State, Zip Code, Telephone)

_____

(Name, Occupation, Address, City, State, Zip Code, Telephone)

Figure 6-7

Completing a Job Application

The job application form provides the employer with the details needed to assess qualifications for employment. It is a personal and professional profile. Use the guidelines provided in the textbook to complete Figure 6-8.

Application for Employment

Date _____

Name _____

Social
Security # _____

Address _____ Zip _____

Telephone
Number _____

If employed and you are under 18 can you furnish a work permit? ☐ Yes ☐ No

Are you legally eligible for employment in the U.S.A.? ☐ Yes ☐ No

Have you worked here before? ☐ Yes ☐ No   If Yes, when? _____

Are there any hours, shifts or days you cannot or will not work? _____

Are you willing to work overtime if required? ☐ Yes ☐ No

List friends or relatives working here. _____

Have you ever been convicted of a crime? ☐ Yes ☐ No (A conviction record will not necessarily be a bar to employment.)

EDUCATION

Circle Highest Grade Completed	Grade School 1 2 3 4 5 6 7 8 High School 9 10 11 12 College 1 2 3 4 Graduate 1 2 3 4	Degree Received	Course Of Study
High School	Name and Address		
College(s)			
Graduate/Professional			
Specialized Training, Apprenticeship, Skills			
Honors and Awards and Accreditations			

MILITARY SERVICE RECORD   Have you served in the U.S. Armed Forces? _____ Dates of duty _____

POSITION(S) APPLIED FOR: 1) _____ 2) _____

You must indicate a specific position. Applications stating "ANY POSITION" will not be considered.

Wage or salary requirements $ _____ When can you start? _____

Figure 6-8

WORK HISTORY

If presently employed, may we contact your employer?　( ) Yes　( ) No

(1) **Present or Most Recent Employer**	Address	Phone
Date Started	Starting Salary	Starting Position
Date Left	Salary on Leaving	Position on Leaving
Name and Title of Supervisor		
Description of Duties		Reason for Leaving
(2) **Previous Employer**	Address	Phone
Date Started	Starting Salary	Starting Position
Date Left	Salary on Leaving	Position on Leaving
Name and Title of Supervisor		
Description of Duties		Reason for Leaving
(3) **Previous Employer**	Address	Phone
Date Started	Starting Salary	Starting Position
Date Left	Salary on Leaving	Position on Leaving
Name and Title of Supervisor		
Description of Duties		Reason for Leaving

Figure 6-8, cont'd

Continued

ADDITIONAL INFORMATION

OTHER QUALIFICATIONS

Summarize special job-related skills and qualifications acquired from employment or other experience.

_____

_____

_____

SPECIALIZED SKILLS   CHECK SKILLS/EQUIPMENT OPERATED

___Keyboarding 45 wpm   ___Fax   Other (list):

___PC   ___Microsoft Office, MedSoft,   _____
                                Altapoint EMR

___Calculator   ___CPR Certification   _____

                             ___Fluent in Spanish   _____

State any additional information you feel may be helpful to us in considering your application. _____

_____

_____

_____

Note to Applicants: DO NOT ANSWER THIS QUESTION UNLESS YOU HAVE BEEN
INFORMED ABOUT THE REQUIREMENTS OF THE JOB FOR WHICH YOU ARE APPLYING.

Are you capable of performing in a reasonable manner, with or without a reasonable accommodation, the activities involved in the job or occupation for which you have applied? A description of the activities involved in such a job or occupation is attached.   ___YES   ___NO

REFERENCES

1. _____   (   ) _____
                              (Name)   Phone #

   _____
                              (Address)

2. _____   (   ) _____
                              (Name)   Phone #

   _____
                              (Address)

3. _____   (   ) _____
                              (Name)   Phone #

   _____
                              (Address)

Under Maryland law, an employer may not require or demand, as a condition of employment, prospective employment, or continued employment, that an individual submit to or take a lie detector or similar test. An employer who violates this law is guilty of a misdemeanour and subject to a fine not exceeding $100.00. By my signature below I certify that I have read the above and understand it completely.

_____   _____
Signature   Date

Figure 6-8, cont'd

Completing an Interview

Use Boxes 6-8, 6-9, and 6-10 in the textbook to conduct a mock interview for a position. Reverse the roles or present your evaluation of the prospective employee as directed by the instructor. Write a summary of the reasons why you would or would not hire the person you interviewed.

Completing a Personal Portfolio

Assemble a portfolio using the HOSA criteria: www.hosa.org/natorg/sectb/cat-v/nrp.pdf

_____ Letter of introduction
_____ Résumé
_____ Project description
_____ Writing sample
_____ Work-based learning
_____ Oral presentation
_____ Community service
_____ Credentials
_____ Technology
_____ Leadership experience

CRITICAL THINKING

Employment Survey

Each student in the class should conduct an interview with an employer to determine which characteristics are most important in an employee. Compile the class information to create a survey form or questionnaire that might be used by an employer to help select incoming employees.

Employment Decisions

Employment decisions are made by supervisors to improve the service provided to the clients by an organization. In health care, this means improving the quality of care given to patients. Use your personal, school, and work experience to explain each of the following decisions.

Questions

1. The employer keeps an employee who always does a minimal job on staff. Another employee, who does a much better job but who has a poor attendance record, is fired.

   _____

   _____

   _____

2. The employer gives a promotion to an employee with less experience than others. The employee who is promoted has a higher level of education for the job.

   _____

   _____

   _____

3. The employer promotes a person with more experience than others. The employee who is promoted has a lower level of education for the job.

   _____

   _____

   _____

4. The employer tells an employee that the work is not being completed in a satisfactory manner. Describe how the employee can handle this situation in a positive manner?

_____

_____

_____

INTERNET ACTIVITIES

Employment Opportunities

Use the Internet to explore the local job opportunities in the occupation of your choice. The national statistics for many occupations may be found on the Occupational Outlook Handbook (OOH) website: http://www.bls.gov/oco

If the career is not included in the OOH website, use a search engine to find the professional organization that represents it.

Key Terms: *occupation, career, information, your career choice*

As directed by your teacher, write a paragraph that describes the career of your choice.

_____

_____

_____

_____

_____

_____

_____

_____

_____

HOSA Site Search

Use the Internet to complete the following questions about HOSA: http://www.hosa.org/

1. What are two national organizations that endorse HOSA?

_____

_____

2. What is one of the new events in the HOSA competition?

_____

3. What is the difference between the Leadership Academy and National Conference?

_____

_____

_____

4. Who is eligible to apply for a HOSA scholarship?

_____

5. What is the current National Theme?

_____

_____

6. What type of information can be found in the HOSA e-magazine?

_____

_____

7. List five of the events that take place during a National Conference.

_____

_____

8. What are HOSA Partnerships?

_____

_____

9. What is found in the HOSA Career Center?

_____

_____

10. How many members does the Executive Council have?

_____

Career Link Inventory

Complete the online Career Link inventory. Write a summary of the information that results. Explain why you agree or disagree with the results.

http://www.mpcfaculty.net/CL/cl.htm

_____

_____

_____

_____

_____

_____

_____

_____

_____

_____

_____

_____

_____

_____

_____

_____

_____

_____

VAPID VOCABULARY

Complete the crossword puzzle using the Key Terms.

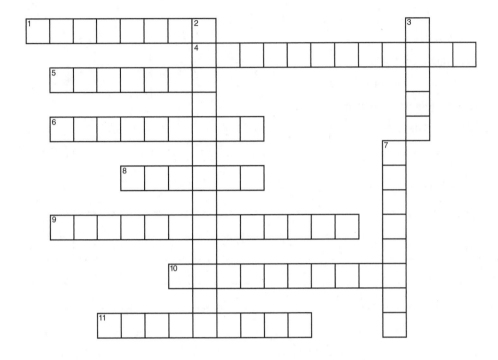

ACROSS

1 Blood pressure during ventricular contraction
4 Act of listening for sounds within the body
5 Whole number, positive or negative and zero
6 Technique used to feel the texture, size, consistency, and location of parts of the body with the hands
8 Pertaining to the apex or pointed end of the heart
9 Pressure of circulating blood against the walls of the arteries (two words)
10 Technique of tapping with the fingertips to evaluate size, borders, and consistency of internal structures of the body
11 Blood pressure during ventricular relaxation

DOWN

2 Sudden stopping of heart action (two words)
3 Necessary to life
7 Number that can be shown as an integer or fraction

ABBREVIATIONS

Match each of the following abbreviations with the phrase that best describes its meaning or function.

Abbreviation	Meaning or Function
1. _____ BP	a. Computer memory
2. _____ I & O	b. Every day
3. _____ NPO	c. Every four hours
4. _____ PDA	d. Force of blood
5. _____ q4h	e. Four times a day
6. _____ qd	f. Handheld computer
7. _____ qid	g. Heat, heart, and breath rate
8. _____ RAM	h. Measurement of food and waste
9. _____ SI	i. Metric system
10. _____ TPR	j. Nothing by mouth

1. BP: _____

2. I & O: _____

3. NPO: _____

4. PDA: _____

5. q4h: _____

6. qd: _____

7. qid: _____

8. RAM: _____

9. SI: _____

10. TPR: _____

JUST THE FACTS

1. The basic health assessment may include an _ _ _ _ _ _ _ _ _ and a
   _ _ ◯ _ _ _ _ _ examination to determine functional, cultural, spiritual, and physical characteristics.

2. The initial patient interview may include the health _ _ ◯ _ _ _ _, nature of the current
   ◯ _ _ _ _ _ _ _ _ _, and medical record.

3. Blood pressure is a measurement of the force of the blood _ _ _ _ _ ◯ _ the walls of the
   _ _ _ _ _ _ _ ◯ as it circulates through the body.

4. Temperature is the measurement of the balance between the heat _ _ _ _ _ _ _ _ and
   _ _ _ ◯ by the body.

5. Pulse is the heartbeat that can be felt (_ _ _ _ _ _ _ _) on surface arteries as the artery walls expand.

62

6. One respiration includes the _ _ _ _ _ _ _ _ _ _ ◯ _ and
_ _ _ ◯ _ _ _ _ _ _ of a breath.

7. Physical assessment uses techniques of inspection, _ _ _ _ _ ◯ _ _ _ _ _ _, palpation,
and _ _ _ _ _ _ _ _ ◯ _ _.

8. Three systems of measurement used in health care are the _ _ ◯ _ _ _ ◯ _ _ _, SI (metric),
and _ _ _ _ _ _ _ _ ◯ units.

9. Computers are used in all aspects of health care, including laboratory tests and
_ _ _ _ ◯ _ _ _ _ _ _ _ _ _ _ _ _ _ _ ◯ _ _ _ _.

10. The purpose of first aid is to sustain ◯ _ _ _ and _ _ _ _ _ _ _ ◯ death.

Use the circled letters to form the answer to this jumble. Clue: What are the two measurements made when taking a blood pressure?

_ _ _ _ _ _ _ _ and _ _ _ _ _ _ _ _ _

CONCEPT APPLICATIONS

Medical Terminology—Fill in the Blank
Use the following prefixes, roots, and suffixes to make and define medical terms.

WORD PART	WORD PART	WORD	MEANING
laparo	otomy		Incision into the abdomen
	ectomy	pneumonectomy	Removal of the lung
hemo	gram	hemogram	
thorax			Incision into the chest
	itis		Inflammation of a clot
path			One who studies disease
pept	ic		
oto	itis		
tympano		tympanitis	
phob	ia		

Medical Terminology—Matching

Match each of the following medical terms with the correct meaning:

Term	Meaning
_____ 1. adenoma	a. Examination of the rectum
_____ 2. arthritis	b. Inflammation of the intestines
_____ 3. cardiology	c. Inflammation of the joints
_____ 4. enteritis	d. Inflammation of the gums
_____ 5. gingivitis	e. Pertaining to organs
_____ 6. mycology	f. Picture of the bone marrow
_____ 7. myelogram	g. Study of fungus
_____ 8. neurology	h. Study of nerves
_____ 9. proctoscopy	i. Study of the heart
_____10. visceral	j. Tumor of a gland

Practicing Math

Complete the following problems using Boxes 7-4 and 7-5 in the textbook. Show your work in the space provided.

1. Determine your body mass index.

2. If a tablet contains 750 mg, how many grams will the patient take if the tablet is broken into two parts?

3. Only caplets of 250 mg of a medication are on hand. If the patient order calls for 0.5 grams of the medication, how many caplets should the patient take?

4. On hand you have a medication in caplet dosages of 50 mg, 0.25 g, and 0.125 mg. The patient order calls for 750 mg. What combination of the medications available would require the fewest caplets?

5. If the patient states that he usually weighs 82 kg, how many pounds does he weigh?

Graphing Practice

Gather and chart the following data.

1. Height of each student in class in centimeters: Chart the data as a line graph using the height as the independent variable and the number of students of that height as the dependent variable.

2. Age of each student in months: Chart the data as a bar graph using the age as the independent variable and the number of students of that age as the dependent variable.

3. Blood pressure and pulse rate of each student in class: Choose a charting method that could be used to compare the blood pressure values in the class with the pulse rates.

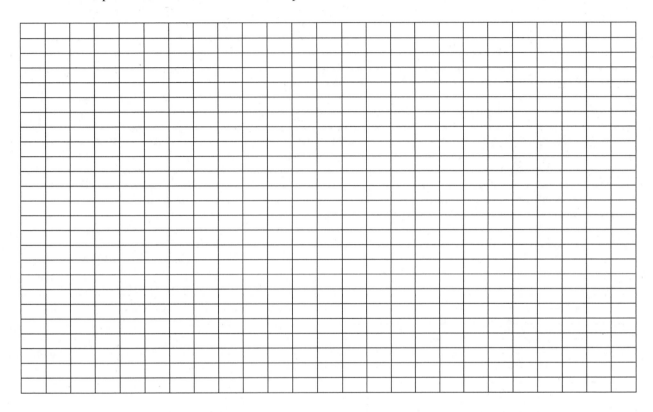

Chapter **7** **Foundation Skills**

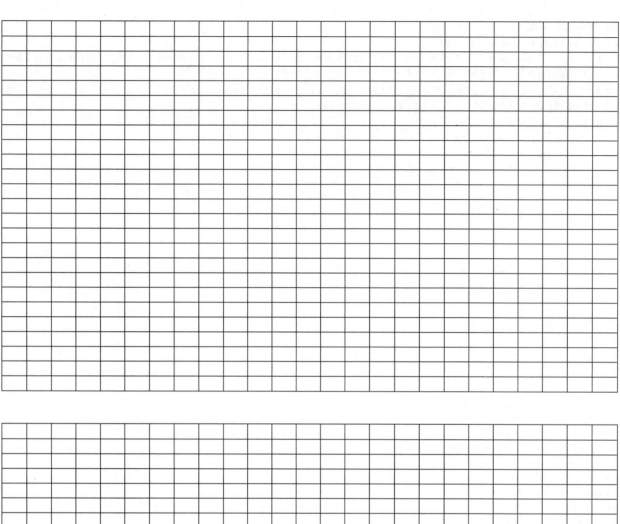

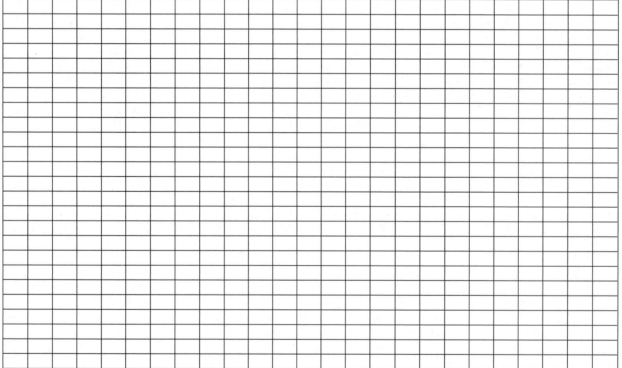

Questions

1. Using the graph, what can you conclude, if anything, about the height of people in your class?

_____

_____

2. Using the graph, what can you conclude, if anything, about the age of people in your class?

_____

_____

3. Using the graph, what can you conclude, if anything, about the relationship of a person's blood pressure and pulse rate?

_____

_____

Physician Orders—Practice

Write directions as described using medical abbreviations.

1. Complete blood count, including hemoglobin and hematocrit

2. Chest x-ray after electrocardiogram

3. Vital signs every 4 hours with weight and height

Conducting an Admission Assessment

Conduct an admission assessment of a fellow student using Figure 7-1.

ADMISSION NURSING ASSESSMENT
STATUS UPON ADMISSION

Admission Notes

Date of admission ___ / ___ / ___   Time _____ a.m. / p.m.

Transported by _____

Accompanied by _____

Age _____ Sex _____ Weight _____ Height: _____ Ft. _____ In.

Vitals: T _____ P _____ (☐ Reg ☐ Irreg) R _____ B/P _____

Attending physician notified? ☐ No ☐ Yes, date/time ___ / ___ / ___ _____ a.m. / p.m.

Diagnosis: _____ Date last chest x-ray or PPD ___ / ___ / ___

Allergies

Meds _____

Food _____

Other _____

Skin Condition

Using the diagrams provided, indicate all body marks such as old/recent scars (surgical and other), bruises, discolorations, abrasions, pressure ulcers, or questionable markings. Indicate size, depth (in cms), color and drainage.

COMMENTS: _____

SPECIAL TREATMENTS & PROCEDURES: _____

PAIN
(As described by resident/representative)

Frequency:
☐ No pain
☐ Less than daily
☐ Daily, but not constant
☐ Constant

Location: _____

Intensity:
☐ No pain
☐ Mild pain
☐ Distressing pain
☐ Severe pain
☐ Horrible pain
☐ Excruciating pain

Pain on admission:
☐ No ☐ Yes, describe _____

RIGHT   LEFT

CURRENT STATUS

General Skin Condition

Check all that apply.
☐ Reddened ☐ Pale ☐ Jaundiced
☐ Cyanotic ☐ Ashen
☐ Dry ☐ Moist ☐ Oily ☐ Warm ☐ Cold
☐ Edema, site _____

Physical Status (describe if applicable otherwise indicate NA)

Paralysis/paresis-site, degree _____
Contracture(s)-site, degree _____
Congenital anomalies _____
Prosthesis: _____
Other _____

Functional Status

TRANSFERS-ABLE TO TRANSFER
☐ Independently
☐ 1 person assist
☐ 2 person assist
☐ Total assist

WEIGHT BEARING-ABLE TO BEAR
☐ Full weight
☐ Partial weight
☐ Non-weight bearing

AMBULATION-ABLE TO AMBULATE
☐ Independently
☐ 1 person assist
☐ 2 person assist
☐ With device
   Type _____
☐ Wheelchair only
☐ Wheelchair/propels self
☐ Bedrest

SUPPORTIVE DEVICES USED:
☐ Elastic hose ☐ Footboard
☐ Bed cradle ☐ Air mattress
☐ Sheepskin ☐ Eggcrate
☐ Hand rolls ☐ Sling ☐ Trapeze
☐ Other _____
☐ Other _____

Drug Therapy

DRUG	DOSE/FREQUENCY	DRUG	DOSE/FREQUENCY
1		6	
2		7	
3		8	
4		9	
5		10	

NAME–Last	First	Middle	Attending Physician	Record No.	Room/Bed

CFS 5-3HH © 1992 Briggs Corporation, Des Moines, IA 50306 (800) 247-2343 PRINTED IN U.S.A.
R1001

ADMISSION NURSING ASSESSMENT
☐ Continued on Reverse

Figure 7-1 (Courtesy of Briggs Corp., Des Moines, Iowa. In Sorrentino SA: *Mosby's Textbook for Nursing Assistants,* ed 7, St Louis, 2008, Mosby/Elsevier.)

Hearing	Right	Left	R & L	Vision	Right	Left	R & L	Communication
Adequate				Adequate				❏ Clear
Adequate w/aid				Adequate w/glasses				❏ Aphasic ❏ Dysphasic
Poor				Poor				Language(s) Spoken:
Deaf				Blind				

Oral Assessment / Eating/Nutrition

Complete oral cavity exam: ❏ Yes ❏ No
If yes, condition _____
_____

Own teeth: ❏ Yes ❏ No
If yes, condition _____

Dentures: Upper ❏ Comp ❏ Part
Lower ❏ Comp ❏ Part
Do dentures fit? ❏ Yes ❏ No

❏ Dependent ❏ Independent ❏ Needs assist

❏ Dysphagic; reason _____

❏ Adaptive equipment (specify) _____
_____

Type/consistency of diet _____
_____

Food likes _____

Food dislikes _____

Bev. preference _____

HS snack preferred: ❏ Yes ❏ No

Sleep Patterns

Usual bed time _____ a.m./p.m.
Usual arising time _____ a.m./p.m.
Usual nap time _____ a.m./p.m.
Other _____

Bathing/Oral Hyg.	Indep.	Assist	Dep.	General Grooming	Indep.	Assist	Dep.
Tub				Shave			
Shower				Grooming			
Bed bath				Dressing			
Oral hygiene				Shampoo			

Psychosocial Functioning

FAMILY RELATIONSHIPS:
Members visit (frequency) _____
_____
Closest relationship with _____
_____
_____

ORIENTED: ❏ Yes ❏ No, if No:
DISORIENTED TO: ❏ Time ❏ Place
❏ Person
RESIDENT GIVEN EXPLANATION OF/OR INVOLVED IN PLAN OF CARE? ❏ Yes ❏ No
RESIDENT ORIENTED TO FACILITY? ❏ Call light ❏ Bathroom ❏ Mealtime ❏ Activities

WHICH WORDS BEST DESCRIBE RESIDENT? ❏ Alert ❏ Angry ❏ Fearful
❏ Noisy ❏ Friendly ❏ Cooperative ❏ Lethargic ❏ ____
❏ Non-questioning ❏ Combative
ANSWERS QUESTIONS: ❏ Readily ❏ Reluntantly ❏ Inappropriately
MOOD: ❏ Passive ❏ Depressed ❏ Elated ❏ Quiet ❏ Secure
❏ Questioning ❏ Talkative ❏ Homesick ❏ Wanders mentally
❏ Hyperactive ❏ ____
COMPREHENSION: ❏ Slow ❏ Quick ❏ Unable to understand
MOTIVATION: ❏ Good ❏ Fair ❏ Poor
PERSONAL HABITS: Smokes? ❏ Yes ❏ No Uses alcohol? ❏ Yes ❏ No

Bowel and Bladder Evaluation

Uses: ❏ Toilet ❏ Urinal ❏ Bedpan ❏ Bedside commode
BOWEL HABITS: Continent? ❏ Yes ❏ No Constipated? ❏ Yes ❏ No Laxative used? ❏ Yes ❏ No
Enemas used? ❏ Yes ❏ No Last bowel movement _____ a.m./p.m.
BLADDER HABITS: Continent? ❏ Yes ❏ No Dribbles? ❏ Yes ❏ No Catheter? ❏ Yes, type _____ ❏ No
Urine color _____ Consistency _____ Time last voiding _____ a.m./p.m.

Restorative Programs Indicated / Therapy Indicated

Based on the foregoing assessment, check all that apply.

❏ ROM
❏ Splint or brace assistance
❏ Bed mobility training & skill practice
❏ Transfer training & skill practice
❏ Walking training & skill practice

❏ Dressing/grooming training & skill practice
❏ Eating/swallowing training & skill practice
❏ Appliance/prosthesis training & skill practice
❏ Communication training & skill practice
❏ Scheduled tolieting
❏ Bladder retraining

❏ Physical
❏ Occupational
❏ Speech
Comments: _____
_____
_____
_____
_____

Comments: _____
_____

Completed by:
Signature/Title _____ Date _____

NAME-Last	First	Middle	Attending Physician	Record No.	Room/Bed

ADMISSION NURSING ASSESSMENT

Figure 7-1 cont'd

Questions

1. Are all of the values you obtained within the normal parameters?

_____

_____

2. If any of the values are abnormal, how could the value be improved?

_____

_____

CRITICAL THINKING

Analyzing Data

Use the following statistics from the Centers for Disease Control website to make a bar graph of the age-adjusted risk factors for heart disease for adults 18-20 years and older. Use the graph to answer the questions.

Data from http://www.cdc.gov/heartDisease/statistics.htm

- Percentage of persons age 20 years and older with hypertension or taking hypertension medications: 32.1%
- Percentage of persons age 20 years and older with high blood cholesterol: 16.9%
- Percentage of persons age 20 years and older with physician-diagnosed diabetes: 10.0%
- Percentage of persons age 20 years and older who are obese: 32.0%
- Percentage of adults age 18 years and older who are current cigarette smokers (2004-2006): 18.4%
- Percentage of adults age 18 years and older who engage in no leisure-time physical activity (2006): 39.5%

Questions

1. What do the data show as the most significant risk factor for developing a heart attack?

_____

2. For which factors are you at risk?

_____

_____

3. Visit the website, http://www.cdc.gov/heartDisease/statistics.htm, and describe one other set of statistics that you find there.

_____

_____

INTERNET ACTIVITIES

Disease Risk

Use the Internet to complete the Siteman Cancer Center disease risk survey for health disease.
  http://www.yourdiseaserisk.wustl.edu/

Questions

1. What is your level of risk for developing heart disease?

_____

2. What tips were you given to prevent the development of heart disease?

_____

_____

_____

Complete at least one of the other risk surveys from the Siteman Cancer Center.

Questions

1. Which risk survey did you select?

_____

2. What is your level of risk for developing the disease?

_____

3. What tips were you given to prevent the development of the disease?

_____

_____

_____

Chapter **7** **Foundation Skills**

Wellness, Growth, and Development

VAPID VOCABULARY

Complete the crossword puzzle using the Key Terms.

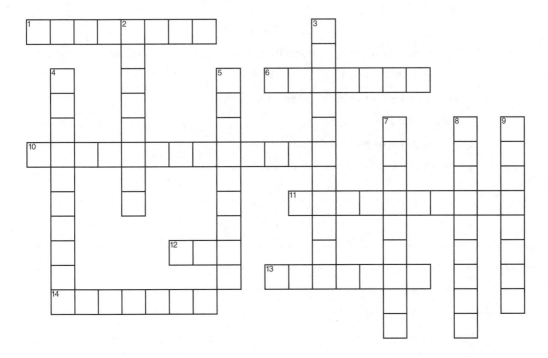

ACROSS

1 Organic compounds needed by the body for metabolism, growth, and development
6 Group of complex organic compounds that are the main part of cell protoplasm
10 Starches, sugars, cellulose, and gums
11 Sum of all the physical and chemical processes by which living organized substance is produced, maintained, and transformed to produce energy
12 Adipose tissue; reserve supply of energy
13 Unit of heat
14 Nonorganic solid substance

DOWN

2 Overdose, 10 times the recommended dose
3 Pearly, fatlike steroid alcohol found in animal fats and oils; precursor of bile acids and hormones
4 Breaking-down process by which complex substances are converted by living cells into simple compounds
5 Proteins, carbohydrates, fats, vitamins, and minerals necessary for growth, normal functioning, and maintaining life
7 Any constructive process by which simple substances are converted by living cells into more complex compounds
8 Dependence on some habit; may be physical, psychological, or both
9 Illness or injury for which there is no reasonable expectation of recovery

ABBREVIATIONS

Match each of the following abbreviations with the phrase that best describes its meaning or function. Then write the phrase or name for each of the abbreviations in the spaces provided.

Abbreviation	Meaning or Function
1. _____ BMI	a. Amount of a nutrient needed daily
2. _____ cal	b. Amount of energy needed to raise 1 gram of water 1 degree centigrade
3. _____ CHO	c. Behavioral model
4. _____ chol	d. Fatlike substance found in animal fats and oils
5. _____ cl liq	e. Government agency that provides leadership on agriculture and natural resources
6. _____ HBM	f. Measurement of body fat
7. _____ kg	g. Measurement of weight (2.2 pounds)
8. _____ RDA	h. Nutrient used for quick energy
9. _____ RDI	i. Nutrient value of processed foods
10. _____ USDA	j. Therapeutic diet that replaces body fluids

1. BMI: _____

2. cal: _____

3. CHO: _____

4. chol: _____

5. cl liq: _____

6. HBM: _____

7. kg: _____

8. RDA: _____

9. RDI: _____

10. USDA: _____

JUST THE FACTS

1. Wellness may be defined as a state of _ _ _ _ _ _ on a continuum from a level of high energy and feeling of well-being to _ _ _ _ _ _ _ or _ _ _ _ _.

2. Fitness may be evaluated by considering muscle strength and endurance, cardiorespiratory _ _ _ _ _ _ _ _ _ _, body _ _ _ _ _ _ _ _ _ _ _, and _ _ _ _ _ _ _ _ _ _ _.

3. Body cells _ _ _ _ _ _ _ _ _ or process food in two ways, called anabolism and _ _ _ _ _ _ _ _ _ _.

4. The five nutrients that have been identified as essential to the maintenance of good health are carbohydrates, _ _ _ _ _ _ _ _, fats, vitamins, and _ _ _ _ _ _ _ _.

5. _ _ _ _ _ _ _ _ _ _ _ _ _ are found in all plants that are used as food sources and are the main source of quick or immediate energy used by the body.

6. In addition to meats, sources of _ _ _ _ _ _ _ ◯ _ include dried beans, peas, and cheese.

7. _ ◯ _ _ are found in the marbling or white part of meat and in cooking oils, salad dressings, and some milk products, such as butter.

8. Stress is the body's _ _ _ _ _ _ _ _ _ _ _ ◯ reaction to the demands of everyday life.

9. _ _ _ _ _ ◯ refers to the changes that can be measured in height, weight, and body proportions, whereas _ _ _ _ _ _ _ _ _ _ _ describes the stages of change in psychological and social functioning.

10. Five stages of dying are _ _ ◯ _ _ _, anger, bargaining, _ _ _ _ _ ◯ _ _ _ _, and acceptance

Use the circled letters to form the answer to this jumble. Clue: What are two of the common physical disorders linked to stress?

_ _ _ _ _ _ _ _ and _ _ _ _ _ _ _ _

CONCEPT APPLICATIONS

Comparing Nutritional Value

With the current food labeling legislation, the consumer has the opportunity to compare the nutritional values of foods as well as the prices. Use the labels in Figure 8-1 to answer the following questions.

Nutrition Facts		
Serving Size 1/2 cup (114 g)		
Servings Per Container 4		
Amount Per Serving		
Calories 90	Calories from Fat 30	
	% Daily Value*	
Total Fat 3 g	5 %	
Saturated Fat 0 g	0 %	
Cholesterol 0 mg	0 %	
Sodium 300 mg	13 %	
Total Carbohydrate 13 g	4 %	
Dietary Fiber 3 g	12 %	
Sugars 3 g		
Protein 3 g		
Vitamin A	80 %	Vitamin C 60 %
Calcium	4 %	Iron 4 %

*Percent daily values are based on a 2000 calorie diet

	Calories	2000	2500
Total Fat	Less than	65 g	80 g
Sat Fat	Less than	20 g	25 g
Cholesterol	Less than	300 mg	300 mg
Sodium	Less than	2400 mg	2400 mg
Total Carbohydrate		300 mg	375 mg
Fiber		25 mg	30 mg

Calories per gram:
Fat 9   Carbohydrate 4   Protein 4

Nutrition Facts		
Serving Size 1 bag (56 g)		
Servings Per Container 1		
Amount Per Serving		
Calories 330	Calories from Fat 250	
	% Daily Value*	
Total Fat 29 g	45 %	
Saturated Fat 3 g	14 %	
Cholesterol 0 mg	0 %	
Sodium 5 mg	0 %	
Total Carbohydrate 10 g	3 %	
Dietary Fiber 4 g	15 %	
Sugars 3 g		
Protein 11 g		
Vitamin A	** %	Vitamin C ** %
Calcium	15 %	Iron 15%

**Less than 2% of Daily Value
*Percent daily values are based on a 2000 calorie diet

	Calories	2000	2500
Total Fat	Less than	65 g	80 g
Sat Fat	Less than	20 g	25 g
Cholesterol	Less than	300 mg	300 mg
Sodium	Less than	2400 mg	2400 mg
Total Carbohydrate		300 mg	375 mg
Fiber		25 mg	30 mg

Calories per gram:
Fat 9   Carbohydrate 4   Protein 4

Figure 8-1

Chapter **8**   **Wellness, Growth, and Development**

Questions

1. Why would one of the food items be better for a person with high blood pressure?

_____

_____

_____

2. Which one of the food items has the best balance of food sources?

_____

_____

_____

3. Which one of the food items would provide a quick source of energy?

_____

_____

_____

4. Explain how a consumer can use the labeling system to determine the amount of calories in the full container of each of the food items shown.

_____

_____

_____

INVESTIGATIONS

Read all directions before beginning this activity. Visit a grocery store to examine labels on food products. Identify five food products that contain at least 50%, by weight, of each of the nutrients in Table 8-1. Record the names of the foods in the spaces provided.

TABLE 8-1   Items Containing 50% of Nutrient by Weight

NUTRIENT	FOOD SOURCE
Protein	
Carbohydrate	
Fat	

Identify five food products that contain at least 50% of the daily value of each of the specified nutrients in Table 8-2. Record the names of the foods in the spaces provided.

Evaluate your list to answer the questions.

TABLE 8-2   Items Containing 50% of Daily Value of Nutrient

NUTRIENT	FOOD SOURCE
Total fat	
Sodium	
Total carbohydrate	
Protein	
Calcium	
Iron	
Vitamin A	
Vitamin C	
Thiamine	
Niacin	
Folic acid	

Questions

1. Which items contain the most minerals? To which food group do they belong?

_____

_____

_____

2. Which items contain the most vitamins? To which food group do they belong?

_____

_____

_____

3. Which items contain the most fat? To which food group do they belong?

_____

_____

_____

Assessing Physical Fitness

Physical fitness is the ability to carry out daily tasks easily and to have enough energy to respond to unexpected demands as necessary. Complete each of the four activities to assess your level of physical fitness. Read all of the directions before beginning this activity. Laboratory activities should be completed under the supervision of a qualified professional only.

Background Information

Components of Physical Fitness

1. Flexibility—Range of movement of joints
2. Strength—Greatest amount of work muscles can do in a given period of time
3. Endurance—How well muscles can perform over a time without causing fatigue
4. Cardiovascular endurance—Ability of the heart and lungs to deliver oxygen to the body during exercise and then quickly to return to a resting rate

DATA CHARTS

Body Flexibility (score in inches)

MEN	WOMEN	RATING
22+	23+	Excellent
17-21	20-22	Good
13-16	17-19	Average
9-12	14-16	Fair
8 or less	13 or less	"Oops"

Leg Muscle Strength
EXCELLENT: A score 5 to 6 inches greater than your height
GOOD: A score 2 to 4 inches greater than your height
FAIR: A score equal to your own height
POOR: A score less than your own height

Muscle Endurance (number of sit-ups in 1 minute)

MEN	WOMEN	RATING
40+	30+	Excellent
33-39	25-29	Good
29-32	18-24	Average
21-28	11-17	Fair
Less than 21	Less than 11	"Oops"

Pulse Recovery Rate (number of heartbeats at the end of 3 minutes of step testing)

PULSE RATE	RATING
70-80	Excellent
81-105	Good
106-119	Average
120-130	Fair
131+	"Oops"

Equipment and Supplies
❑ Mat or blanket
❑ Stepladder or heavy box
❑ Stopwatch or watch with a second hand
❑ Tape measure or meter stick

Instructions

Activity 1—Flexibility
1. Do some light stretching exercises to warm up your muscles and to prevent injury.
2. Avoid quick, jerking movements. Use gradual, smooth movements.
3. Sit on the floor with your legs straight in front of you. Your heels should be 5 inches apart.
4. Place a yardstick on the floor with the 36-inch mark pointing away from your body. The 15-inch mark should be even with your heels.
5. Slowly reach with both hands as far forward as possible and hold the position.
6. Measure the most distant point that the fingertips reach.
7. Repeat twice more for a total of three trials.

Activity 2—Leg Muscle Strength
1. From the starting point, bend your knees and jump forward (standing broad jump), landing on both feet.
2. Measure your jump in inches.
3. Repeat twice more for a total of three trials.

Activity 3—Muscle Endurance
1. Lie on your back on a mat or blanket with your knees slightly bent. Your partner holds your ankles in place.
2. Place your hands behind your head and perform as many sit-ups as you can do in 1 minute.
3. Take care to breathe freely; do not hold your breath. Return to a flat lying position after each sit-up.
4. Repeat twice more for a total of three trials.

Activity 4—Cardiovascular Endurance
1. Take a resting pulse rate for 1 minute and record it.
2. While your partner supports the stepladder, step up and down (both feet) continuously for 3 minutes.
3. Step at the rate of 24 steps per minute.
4. Immediately sit down at the end of 3 minutes and take your pulse rate for 1 minute.
5. Rest without talking and monitor your pulse every minute. Record the amount of time needed for your heart to return to its resting rate.

TABLE 8-3   Your Results

Activity 1—Flexibility	Result
Trial 1	
Trial 2	
Trial 3	
Activity 2—Leg Muscle Strength	Result
Trial 1	
Trial 2	
Trial 3	
Activity 3—Muscle Endurance	Result
Trial 1	
Trial 2	
Trial 3	
Activity 4—Cardiovascular Endurance	Result
Trial 1	
Trial 2	
Trial 3	

Questions

1. Calculate the average result and determine your rating for each of the activities:

   Activity 1 average _____

   Activity 2 average _____

   Activity 3 average _____

   Activity 4 average _____

2. In which area(s) of physical fitness would you like to improve your performance?

   _____

   _____

   _____

3. What could you do differently in your life to make the improvements listed?

   _____

   _____

   _____

4. What is an aerobic exercise? Give an example of an aerobic exercise.

   _____

   _____

   _____

5. A lifetime sport is one that can be done throughout the life span. Describe at least one lifetime sport in which you participate.

   _____

   _____

   _____

6. "Being active naturally" is a phrase described to include exercise in your daily routine and activities. An example would be to park a distance from the door of the store in order to walk farther to and from the car. Give one example of natural activity in which you participate.

   _____

   _____

   _____

CRITICAL THINKING

Making the Decision to Die

In 1993 Michigan passed a law that makes assisted suicide a felony. This law resulted from the more than 17 assisted suicides involving Dr. Jack Kevorkian. Groups that oppose Dr. Kevorkian's actions question whether all of the suicides were actually voluntary.

When the Oregon Death with Dignity Act was passed in 1994, Oregon became the first state to legalize assisted suicide. However, the law was immediately challenged in the courts. This new legislation allows physicians to assist suicide in cases of terminal illness in which the life expectancy is 6 months or less. To obtain lethal medication under the law, the person must be diagnosed as terminal by at least two physicians. Groups that oppose the measure are concerned that people who are ill will choose to commit suicide to prevent expensive medical bills or to spare their loved ones from providing care for them.

In 1994 Benito Agrelo, a 15-year-old Florida boy, fought in court for the right to refuse a third transplant and medication. Benny had been born with a malfunctioning liver and had previously undergone two liver transplants. The drugs used to keep Benny's body from rejecting the liver caused migraine headaches and severe leg and back pain. Benny could not read or walk. Benny's physicians felt that Benny could be helped by a third transplant and a change in the dosage of the immunosuppressive medication. Using the child abuse agencies and laws, the physicians forced Benny to return to the hospital. After hearings with a judge, Benny was allowed to return home and refuse treatment. Benny stopped taking the medication and died in August 1994. Before he died, he reported that those last months were the best months of his life.

In 2006, 16-year-old Abraham Cherrix went to court in Virginia to win the right to refuse chemotherapy for treatment of Hodgkin disease. Abraham had been previously treated with chemotherapy but chose to follow an alternative treatment when the disease reappeared. His parents were charged with medical negligence. In August, 2006, charges against his parents were dropped when Abraham agreed to treatment by an oncologist who is supportive of the alternative medicine approach.

Questions

1. In your opinion, is it suicide for a person to refuse treatment, as Abraham did, or medication, as in the case of Benny?

_____

_____

_____

2. In your opinion, should someone who is terminally ill be allowed to commit suicide?

_____

_____

_____

3. If you gave a positive response to question 2, who do you think should be involved in a decision to end someone's life?

_____

_____

_____

4. In your opinion, what gives a person's life value?

_____

_____

_____

INTERNET ACTIVITIES

Creating a Food Pyramid

Use the USDA website to create a personal food pyramid:
    http://www.mypyramid.gov/
    http://www.mypyramid.gov/mypyramid/index.aspx

Age: _____

Sex: _____

Physical activity: _____

Grains: _____

Vegetables: _____

Fruits: _____

Milk: _____

Meat and beans: _____

Number of calories required: _____

81

Questions

1. List some of the types of foods you prefer from each of the five food groups.

   a. Grains: _____

   b. Vegetables: _____

   c. Fruits: _____

   d. Milk: _____

   e. Meat and beans: _____

2. Describe things you could do to change your physical activity, if needed.

   _____

   _____

   _____

3. Design a 24-hour meal plan that meets the requirement of your pyramid.

   _____

   _____

   _____

   _____

   _____

   _____

   _____

   _____

   _____

Comparing Types of Fat

Use the Internet to research and complete the following chart about dietary fats.

   Suggested Resources
   Mayo Clinic: http://www.mayoclinic.com/health/fat/NU00262
   Harvard: http://www.hsph.harvard.edu/nutritionsource/what-should-you-eat/fats-and-cholesterol/

Dietary Fats

TYPE OF FAT	FOOD SOURCES	APPEARANCE AT ROOM TEMPERATURE	CONSIDERED HELPFUL OR HARMFUL
Monounsaturated			
Polyunsaturated			
Omega-3 fatty acid			
Saturated			
Trans			

Amino Acids

Use the Internet to research and complete the following questions about amino acids.

Suggested Resources

University of Arizona: http://www.biology.arizona.edu/biochemistry/problem_sets/aa/aa.html

How Stuff Works: http://www.howstuffworks.com/food3.htm

About.com: http://nutrition.about.com/od/basicnutritioncourse/a/eclassprotein.htm

Everyday Diet: http://www.everydiet.org/articles/protein.htm

Questions

1. What are amino acids?

_____

_____

_____

2. What is an essential amino acid?

_____

_____

_____

3. How many essential amino acids are there?

_____

4. List the essential amino acids.

_____

_____

_____

5. Define and give an example of a complete protein.

_____

_____

_____

BMR and Calories

Use the Internet to calculate your basal metabolic rate (BMR) and daily caloric needs. You can use the following website:

Discovery Health - http://health.discovery.com/tools/calculators/basal/basal.html

Myfoodpedia - http://www.myfoodapedia.gov/

Questions

1. How does a person's BMR relate to the individual's daily caloric needs?

_____

_____

_____

2. What factors are considered in figuring the BMR?

_____

_____

_____

3. What is your caloric need to maintain your current weight, as calculated using your BMR?

_____

Balancing Calories in Foods and Activities

A balanced diet provides the recommended number of servings of the five food groups each day. It also contains enough calories to meet the person's energy needs to complete the activities of the day.

Determine the caloric value of the food eaten and the activities performed on the day described, using the Internet to locate calorie charts for food and exercise. Use the information provided in the chapter to evaluate the diet's nutritional value and to answer the questions.

Calories Gained by Eating

Nutricounter: http://www.calorie-counter-chart.com/index.htm
Diet-i.com: http://www.diet-i.com/calorie_chart/fast-food.htm
Mike's Calorie Chart: http://www.ntwrks.com/~mikev/chart1.html

Calories Used Through Exercise

Diet-i.com: http://www.diet-i.com/calorie_table/burgers.htm
Med India: http://www.medindia.net/patients/calculators/calorie_chart.asp

Singsa Blues is a girl, age 16 years, who would like to lose approximately 15 pounds. Singsa weighs 135 pounds and is 5′4″ tall. The following is her usual diet for 1 day. Calculate the number of calories contained in the foods Singsa ate on the day indicated. Enter the information in Table 8-4.

TABLE 8-4

BREAKFAST		LUNCH		DINNER		SNACK	
FOOD	**CALORIES**	**FOOD**	**CALORIES**	**FOOD**	**CALORIES**	**FOOD**	**CALORIES**
1 fried egg		BLT sandwich – 2 slices toast		6 oz steak		1 cup ice cream	
2 slices toast		BLT – 2 slices tomato		½ cup broccoli		1 T chocolate sauce	
3 T jelly		BLT – 3 strips bacon		1 cup potatoes			
1 glass whole milk		BLT – 1 piece lettuce		¼ cup gravy			
1 glass OJ		BLT – 2 T mayonnaise		1 glass whole milk			
		1 can soda					

Singsa usually participates in the following activities each day. Use the Internet to locate calorie and exercise charts to calculate the calories needed to complete the activities in Table 8-5.

TABLE 8-5

ACTIVITY	TIME	CALORIES USED
Dressing and eating breakfast	30 minutes	
Walking to bus stop	5 minutes	
Riding bus 1 mile to school	15 minutes	
Sitting in morning classes	3 hours	
Eating lunch sitting at table	1 hour	
Sitting in afternoon classes	2 hours	
Riding bus home	15 minutes	
Sitting watching TV	2 hours	
Eating dinner	15 minutes	
Sitting doing homework	30 minutes	
Sleeping	9 hours	

Questions

1. What was Singsa's overall calorie intake?

   _____

2. What was Singsa's overall calorie output?

   _____

3. Use the following formula to estimate Singsa's caloric needs if she wishes to maintain a body weight of 120 pounds:

   Weight in pounds × 15 calories per pound per day = Necessary calories per day

   _____ lb × 15 cal/lb/day = _____ cal/day

4. How many servings of each of the five food groups did Singsa eat on this day?

Meat or protein	_____	servings
Milk or equivalent	_____	servings
Fruits	_____	servings
Vegetables	_____	servings
Bread or cereal	_____	servings
Fats	_____	servings

5. Explain why Singsa will gain (or lose) weight on this day.

   _____

   _____

   _____

6. Because 3500 calories equal 1 pound of weight, how would Singsa's diet affect her weight in 1 week if she followed the same meal and activity plan every day?

_____

_____

_____

7. List at least five specific changes Singsa could make to her diet so that she would lose weight while eating the recommended number of servings of the food groups.

_____

_____

_____

8. List five specific changes Singsa could make to her activity routine to help her lose weight.

_____

_____

_____

9. Calculate the number of calories you would need to eat to maintain your desired weight.

_____

_____

_____

9 | Body Organization

VAPID VOCABULARY

Find the key terms in the word search puzzle and define them in the spaces provided.

```
E S Z G L G I S P L J P E X N
M T N M B Z Y H S K U H P M G
T W Y S E N X X I N I E Y M I
A N Z L D S A O S A L N T N N
U A A R O N A Y A A R O O O E
T M O N X R T E T Y C T N R B
O M A X I I T I S T M Y E G B
S X O L D M N C O I C P G A M
O G F E I E O T E U D E N N Y
M R R I G G K D M L J R X I Z
E E K N W X N Y O E E P D S K
H M O T O M U A H L V J C M R
S C J K C T C O N D I T I O N
Q T A I C A G M U T A T I O N
E V I S S E C E R H I M X U T
```

1. Autosome: _____

2. Benign: _____

3. Condition: _____

4. Congenital: _____

5. Disease: _____

6. Dominant: _____

7. Electrolyte: _____

8. Genotype: _____

Continued

9. Heredity: _____

10. Homeostasis: _____

11. Malignant: _____

12. Mutation: _____

13. Organism: _____

14. Phenotype: _____

15. Recessive: _____

16. Syndrome: _____

ABBREVIATIONS

Match each of the following abbreviations with the phrase that best describes its meaning or function. Then write the phrase or name for each of the abbreviations in the spaces provided.

Abbreviation	Meaning or Function
1. _____ CA	a. Agency that regulates vaccinations
2. _____ CF	b. Disorders caused by more than one gene
3. _____ CVS	c. Federal agency that is cataloguing descriptions of genetic disorders
4. _____ DNA	d. Federal project to identify genetic mutations
5. _____ FDA	e. Genetic code
6. _____ HBV	f. Genetic disorder leading to respiratory problems
7. _____ HPV	g. Hepatitis virus
8. _____ MFGD	h. Test used to check DNA of unborn fetus
9. _____ NCBI	i. Uncontrolled cell growth
10. _____ TCGA	j. Virus that causes cervical cancer

1. CA: _____

2. CF: _____

3. CVS: _____

4. DNA: _____

5. FDA: _____

6. HBV: _____

7. HPV: _____

8. MFGD: _____

9. NCBI: _____

10. TCGA: _____

Use the following prefixes, roots, and suffixes to make and define terms related to disorders of body organization.

WORD PART	WORD PART	WORD	MEANING
adeno	oma		Tumor of the gland
blast			Cancer of immature cells
	genic	carcinogenic	Cancer causing
chemo	therapy		Treatment with medication
chondro			Tumor of cartilage
cyto	toxic		Poisonous to cells
derma		dermatitis	Inflammation of the skin
hepati	blastoma	hepatoblastoma	
histo		histologist	
	emia	leukemia	Blood cancer
lympho		lymphoma	
	ectomy	mastectomy	
melano			Skin cancer
	ectomy	nephrectomy	Excision or removal of the kidney
	ology	oncology	
osteo		osteogenic	
		sarcoma	Tumor of connective tissue
path		pathologist	
toxo		toxicology	

1. The four basic properties of life are conception, _ _ _ _ Ⓞ _ _ _ _ _, reproduction, and
   _ _ _ Ⓞ _ _ _ _ _ _ _ _ _.

2. The two major types of study of the human body are called _ _ _ Ⓞ _ _ _ and
   _ _ _ _ _ _ Ⓞ _ _ _.

3. _ _ _ _ _ _ _ Ⓞ _ _ _ is the tendency of a cell or the whole organism to maintain
   a state of balance.

4. The four types of tissue in the body are _ _ _ _ _ _ _ _ Ⓞ _,
   _ _ _ _ _ _ _ _ Ⓞ _, muscle, and nerve.

5. Ⓞ _ _ _ _ _ _ is the process by which a cell divides to reproduce, creating a copy with the same
   chromosomes.

6. In the process of _ _ _ _ _ _ _, the cell divides into two parts, each with only one half of the
   chromosomes.

7. _ _ _ _ _ _ _ Ⓞ is the passing on of genetic information that determines the characteristics of an
   individual person.

8. Abnormal genes or chromosomes cause many disorders, which therefore are called inherited,
   _ _ _ _ Ⓞ _ _ _ _ _, or _ _ _ _ _ _ _ Ⓞ disorders.

9. _ _ Ⓞ _ _ _ is the uncontrolled growth of abnormal cells that tend to spread (metastasize) and invade
   the tissue around them.

10. Three disorders that have been linked to genetic factors include _ _ _ _ _ _ cancer,
    _ _ _ _ Ⓞ _ _ _ _ _ _ _ _ _, and
    _ _ _ _ Ⓞ _ _ _ Ⓞ _ disease.

   Use the circled letters to form the answer to this jumble. Clue: What is the area of the body that contains the stomach,
liver, and spleen?

   _ _ _ _ _ _ _ _ _   _ _ _ _ _ _

Identifying Structures of the Cell

Use Figure 9-1 in the textbook to label and color the diagram of the cell in Figure 9-1. In the spaces provided in Table 9-1, describe the function of each part.

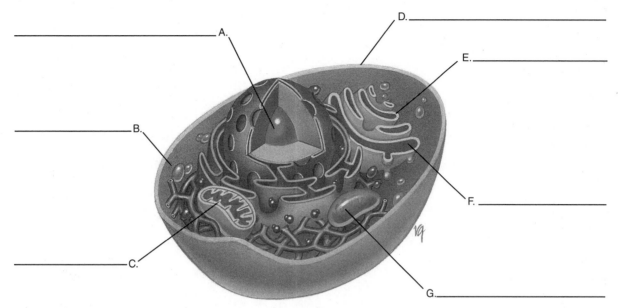

Figure 9-1   (From Patton KT, Thibodeau GA: *Anatomy & physiology,* ed 7, St Louis, 2010, Mosby/Elsevier.)

TABLE 9-1   Functions of the Cell

CELL PART	FUNCTION
Cell membrane	
Cytoplasm	
Golgi apparatus	
Lysosome	
Mitochondria	
Nucleus	
Ribosome	
Smooth endoplasmic reticulum	

Identifying Body Planes

Use Figure 9-5 in the textbook to list the body planes shown in Figure 9-2.

1. _____

2. _____

3. _____

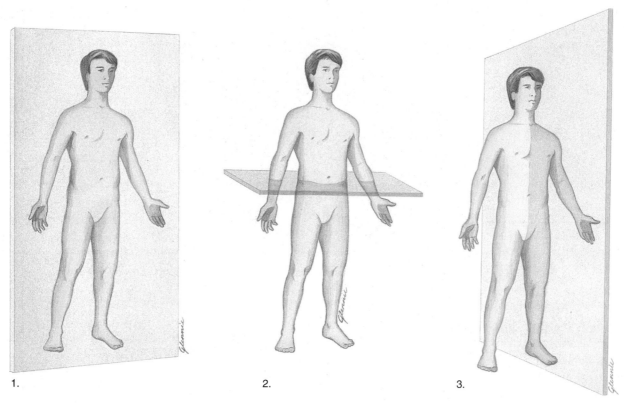

1.   2.   3.

Figure 9-2

Identifying Body Cavities

Use Figure 9-6 in the textbook to label the diagram of the body cavities in Figure 9-3. Shade or color the cavities that are considered to be located on the dorsal side of the body. In the spaces provided in Table 9-2, list at least two organs or structures found in each body cavity.

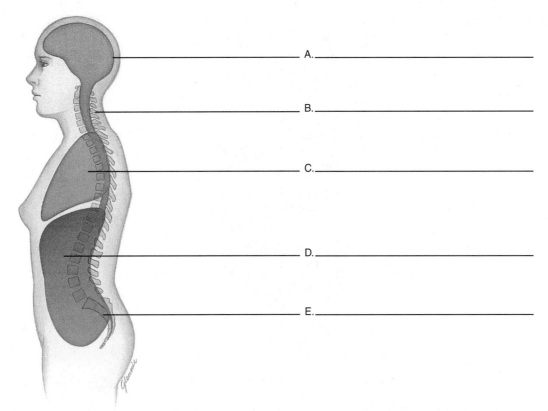

A._____

B._____

C._____

D._____

E._____

Figure 9-3

TABLE 9-2   Body Cavities

BODY CAVITY	STRUCTURES LOCATED IN THE CAVITY
A.	
B.	
C.	
D.	
E.	

Chapter **9   Body Organization**

Identifying Body Regions

Use Figure 9-7 in the textbook to list the body regions shown in Figure 9-4.

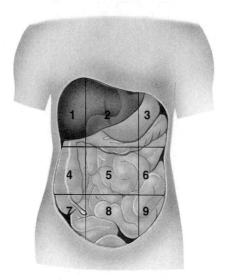

Figure 9-4

1. _____

2. _____

3. _____

4. _____

5. _____

6. _____

7. _____

8. _____

9. _____

Identifying Disorders of Body Organization

Complete the missing information about genetic disorders in Table 9-3 using the textbook chapters indicated in parentheses. Note the etiology (causing factor), signs and symptoms, and treatment and method of prevention (if any).

Applying Your Knowledge

1. Why is a hereditary characteristic referred to as a condition, syndrome, or disorder instead of a disease?

_____

_____

_____

_____

2. The hereditary condition that affects the appearance of the mouth and that can be controlled with plastic surgery is called _____.

3. The condition that may result in myelomeningocele is called _____.

4. The condition that results in too many red blood cells is called _____.

TABLE 9-3   Disorders of Body Organization

DISORDER	ETIOLOGY	SIGNS AND SYMPTOMS	TREATMENT AND PREVENTION
Cleft lip or palate (Chapter 10)			
Clubfoot (Chapter 14)			
Cystic fibrosis (Chapter 13)			
Down syndrome (Chapter 19)			
Huntington disease (Chapter 19)			
Klinefelter's syndrome (Chapter 21)			
Neural tube defect (Chapter 19)			
Neurofibromatosis (Chapter 19)			
Phenylketonuria (Chapter 16)			
Sickle cell anemia (Chapter 12)			
Spina bifida (Chapter 19)			
Tay-Sachs (Chapter 16)			
Thalassemia (Chapter 12)			

Identifying Tissue Types

Read all directions before beginning the activity. Laboratory activities should be performed under the supervision of a qualified professional only.

Equipment and Supplies

Cover slip (optional)
Microscope
Prepared slides of tissue types
Raw chicken wing, blood sample, cheek cells (optional)
Slide (optional)

Directions

1. Review the procedure for using a microscope found in Chapter 22.
2. Observe prepared slides of four types of body tissue under low power and high power.
3. Draw your observations of the four tissue types in the spaces provided in Figure 9-5.
4. Prepare a wet slide using a thin slice of tissue from a raw chicken wing, cheek cells, blood, or other specimen.
5. Identify the tissue type on the slide.
6. Draw your observation in the space provided in Figure 9-5.
7. Return all equipment and supplies to the designated location.

Drawing Conclusions

1. In your opinion, which kind of tissue is the easiest to identify? Why?

   _____

   _____

   _____

2. Which kind of tissue(s) did you observe in the chicken wing sample?

   _____

   _____

   _____

3. In your opinion, which tissue type is the most diverse or has the most varied structures in the body?

   _____

   _____

   _____

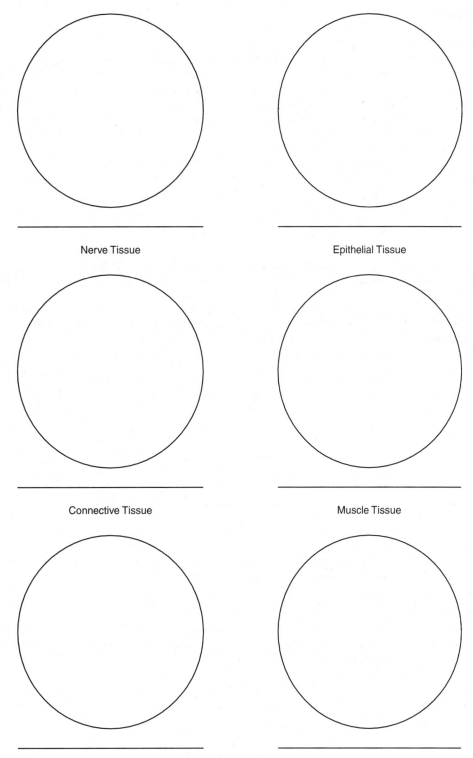

Nerve Tissue

Epithelial Tissue

Connective Tissue

Muscle Tissue

Figure 9-5

Chapter **9** **Body Organization**

Determining Probability of Inheritance

Cystic fibrosis is often used to study hereditary traits because a recessive, autosomal gene carries it. Cystic fibrosis results in the inadequate production of certain enzymes. The condition is characterized by too much mucus in the lungs. It can be detected by testing for salt on the skin. Treatment includes eating a diet that is high in protein and calories. The person with this condition also must use good pulmonary hygiene, which may include postural drainage, to keep the lungs free of excess secretions. Postural drainage involves positioning the body to drain secretions into the bronchi so that they may be removed or excreted by coughing. Antibiotics are used to treat infections if they occur. People with cystic fibrosis may live well past middle age with proper care.

Cystic fibrosis is the most commonly occurring recessive disorder in the white population.

The probability of inheriting a genetic disorder may be determined using a Punnett square. In the example of cystic fibrosis, the parents may have a genetic configuration of genotype as follows:

Father's Genotype   Mother's Genotype
       Ff   Ff

Both parents are carriers. That means that they both carry the recessive gene (f) for cystic fibrosis, but they do not have the condition themselves because the gene is recessive. Having the dominant gene (F) means that the phenotype, or appearance, of each of these individuals is not to have cystic fibrosis.

During meiosis, or sexual cell reproduction, the sperm and egg of the mother and father are formed using one of the genes possible for this trait. The chances of the sperm and egg containing the F or the f gene are exactly equal.

The Punnett square can be used to determine the probability that the offspring will show the condition of cystic fibrosis. The square is formed by placing the father's genes on top and the mother's genes on the side, as shown in Figure 9-6.

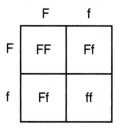

Figure 9-6

The probability of the offspring having the condition of cystic fibrosis (genotype ff) is one in four, or 1/4. The probability of the offspring being a carrier (genotype Ff) is two in four, or 1/2.

Examining the Evidence

1. Complete the Punnett square shown in Figure 9-7 to determine the probability of a couple showing the following genotypes producing an offspring with cystic fibrosis. The father's phenotype is that he has the condition (genotype ff). The mother is a carrier (genotype Ff).

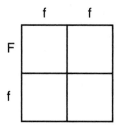

Figure 9-7

The probability of the offspring having cystic fibrosis (genotype ff) is _____ in four, or _____.
The probability of the offspring being a carrier (genotype Ff) is _____ in four, or _____. The probability of the couple producing a child without the condition is _____ in four, or _____.

98

2. Complete the Punnett square in Figure 9-8 for a couple who has the following phenotypes. The father is a carrier (genotype Ff). The mother does not carry this recessive gene (genotype FF).

Figure 9-8

The probability of the offspring having cystic fibrosis (genotype ff) is _____ in four, or _____.
The probability of the offspring being a carrier (genotype Ff) is _____ in four, or _____. The probability of the couple producing a child without the condition is _____ in four, or _____.

3. Why is the probability of the second child showing the condition of cystic fibrosis for the couple in question 1 the same as the probability of their first child having this genetic configuration?

_____

_____

_____

4. Why is the probability of the sperm containing the F or f gene exactly the same when the father's genotype is Ff?

_____

_____

_____

INTERNET ACTIVITIES

Cell Phone Safety

Safety of cell phones and a link to cancer has been debated for several years. The concern comes from the low-level exposure to radio frequency (RF) electromagnetic fields from the phones to the individual's brain.

In 1998 and 1999, fourteen countries participated in a series of case-control studies about the relationship of cell phones to brain cancer. The International Agency for Research on Cancer (IARC) coordinated the study. This was called the INTERPHONE study. In the December 2009 issue of *New Scientist*, the preliminary results of the study were reviewed.

Use the following Internet site to investigate and describe the study findings in a paragraph. What was a common bias of the participants?

Key Terms: INTERPHONE study

New Scientist: http://www.newscientist.com/article/dn18223-cellphones-and-cancer-interphone-cant-end-the-debate.html?full=true

_____

_____

_____

_____

_____

_____

_____

_____

Chapter **9** **Body Organization**

Karyotype Online Simulation

Use the following Internet link to simulate genetic disorders due to karyotype abnormalities. Complete the karyotype for each of the three patients.

University of Arizona Biology Project:
http://www.biology.arizona.edu/human_bio/activities/karyotyping/karyotyping.html

Questions

1. How many karyotype analyses are performed in the United States and Canada each year?

   _____

2. What notation would you use to characterize Patient A's karyotype?

   _____

3. What diagnosis would you give Patient A?

   _____

4. What notation would you use to characterize Patient B's karyotype?

   _____

5. What diagnosis would you give Patient B?

   _____

6. What notation would you use to characterize Patient C's karyotype?

   _____

7. What diagnosis would you give Patient C?

   _____

8. Use the Internet to research and describe in a paragraph the signs and symptoms of one of the disorders.

   _____

   _____

   _____

   _____

   _____

   _____

   _____

   _____

   _____

   _____

10 Integumentary System

Integumentary System

VAPID VOCABULARY

Find the key terms in the word search puzzle and define them in the spaces provided.

```
J D K M Q C J J W D I J L S S
V F E G L E R P N N B Y U E U
I D A R N S W I C I M O S S O
C E R U M I N O U S R E H O E
Z R U C P A L R X E B P L P N
T M X P L U T O F A H I E I A
I I S E N T G I C B D D A D T
R S M U Z T R E T E V E H A U
Z E L V K O O I I I F R A P C
P A I Z D U W B K J S M W K B
K M I U S S U L I P A I Y C U
B K S E L C I L L O F S H Q S
P A P I L L A U D M P L T M D
U B T U J S X J Y O D S S C R
A R R Y H T W N H R R Y Q S
```

1. Adiposes:_____

2. Biopsy: _____

3. Ceruminous:_____

4. Dermatitis:_____

5. Dermis:_____

6. Epidermis: _____

7. Follicle: _____

8. Lunula:_____

9. Melanin: _____

Continued

10. Papilla: _____

11. Pilus: _____

12. Sebaceous: _____

13. Subcutaneous: _____

14. Sudoriferous: _____

ABBREVIATIONS

Match each of the following abbreviations with the phrase that best describes its meaning or function. Then write the phrase or name for each of the abbreviations in the spaces provided.

Abbreviation

1. _____ CDC
2. _____ FDA
3. _____ KS
4. _____ LE
5. _____ mL
6. _____ PABA
7. _____ PDT
8. _____ SPF
9. _____ UV
10. _____ Vit D

Meaning or Function

a. Benign dermatitis that may become a systemic disorder

b. Government agency that monitors contagious disorders

c. Government agency that regulates cosmetics

d. Liquid measurement of water lost by the skin as sweat

e. Measurement of the amount of sun that is blocked

f. Product that blocks harmful rays of the sun

g. Rays of the sun that are harmful to skin cells

h. Treatment that involves injecting drugs into blood vessels around cancer and then exposing the area to light

i. Type of cancer associated with AIDs

j. Vitamin produced in the skin

1. CDC: _____

2. FDA: _____

3. KS: _____

4. LE: _____

5. mL: _____

6. PABA: _____

7. PDT: _____

8. SPF: _____

9. UV: _____

10. Vit D: _____

JUST THE FACTS

1. The skin is the __ __ __ __ __ __ __   __ __ __ __ __ in the body.

2. The three types of glands in the skin are the __ __ __ __ __ __ __ __ __ glands, the
__ __ __ __ __ __ __ __ __ __ __ __ glands, and the __ ◯ __ __ __ __ __ __ __ __ glands.

3. Ceruminous glands are located only in the _ _ _ Ⓞ _ _ _ _ _   _ _ _ _ _ _ of the ear.

4. Skin disorders are usually uncomfortable and unattractive but not

   _ _ _ _ -_ _ _ _ _ _ _ _ _ _ _ _ _ _ _.

5. Acne usually appears in adolescence and often is caused by the _ _ _ Ⓞ _ _ _ _ _
   _ _ _ _ _ _ _ _ _ of oil related to increased hormones during puberty.

6. Two skin disorders that lead to a change in pigmentation include _ _ _ _ _ _ _ _ and

   _ _ _ _ _ _ _ _.

7. Two skin disorders caused by bacteria include _ _ _ _ _ _ _ _ _ _ and
   _ Ⓞ _ _ _ _ _ _.

8. All soaps work by emulsification; they surround and bind to the dirt so that it can be

   _ _ _ _ _ Ⓞ _ _ _ _.

9. The skin defends against the damaging ultraviolet radiation of the sun by producing _ _ _ _ _ _ _.

10. _ _ Ⓞ _ _ _   _ _ _ _ carcinoma is the most common type of skin cancer.

   Use the circled letters to form the answer to this jumble. Clue: What is the layer of the skin that contains the blood and nerve vessels called?

   _ _ _ _ _ _

CONCEPT APPLICATIONS

Identifying Structures of the Skin
Use Figure 10-1 in the textbook to label and color the diagram of the skin in Figure 10-1.

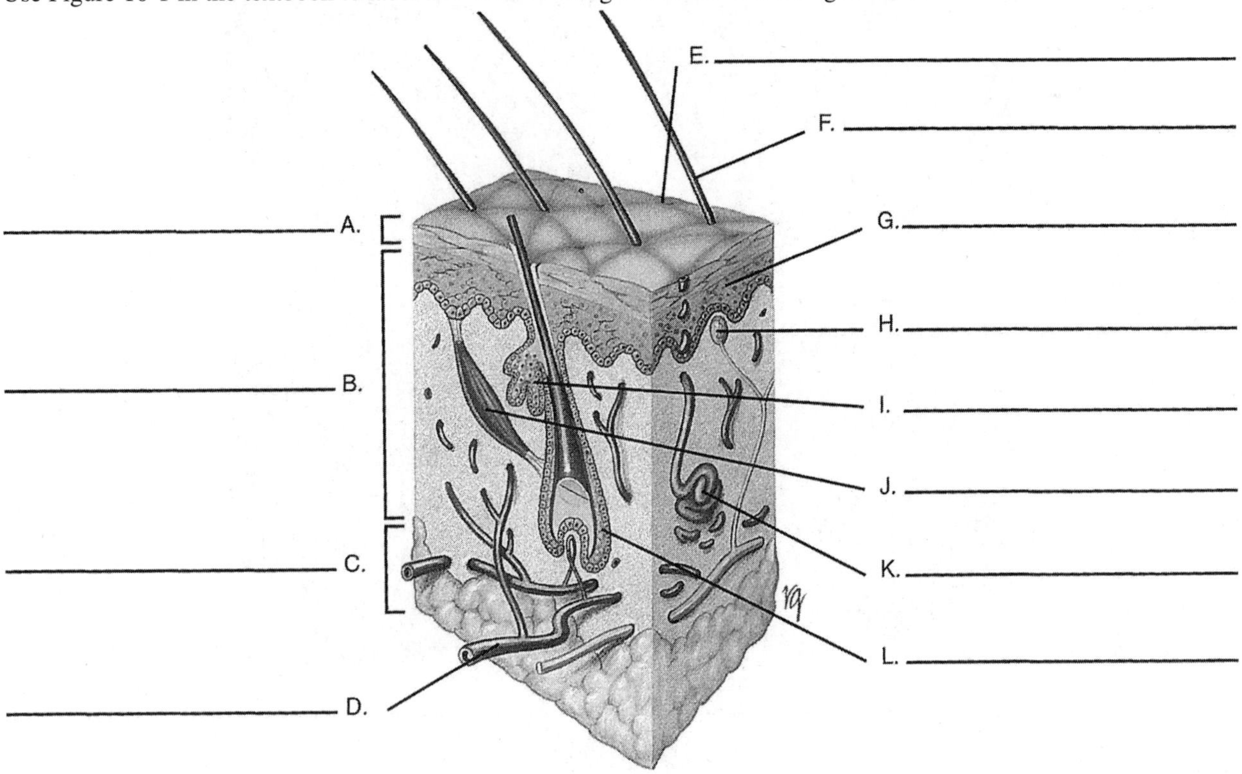

Figure 10-1

Describe the function of each part in Table 10-1.

TABLE 10-1   Functions of the Skin

SKIN PART	MAIN FUNCTION
Arrector pili	
Blood vessel	
Dermis	
Epidermis	
Hair root	
Hair shaft	
Melanocyte	
Nerve cell	
Pore	
Sebaceous gland	
Subcutaneous	
Sudoriferous gland	

Identifying Skin Lesions

Use the Internet and descriptions of skin lesions in Table 10-2 in the textbook to identify the Figure 10-2 diagrams. Identify the possible cause in Table 10-2 of the workbook.

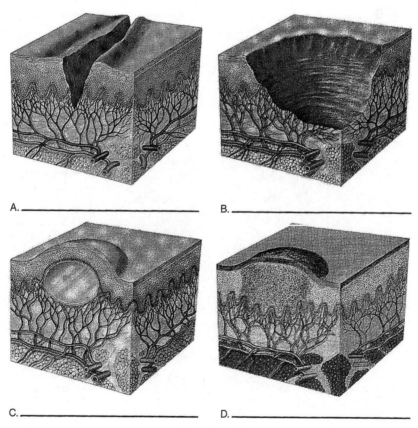

A. _____   B. _____

C. _____   D. _____

Figure 10-2

TABLE 10-2   Causes of Lesions

LESION	CAUSE
Cyst	
Fissure	
Papule	
Ulcer	

Identifying Disorders of the Integumentary System

Use the textbook to complete the missing information about integumentary system disorders in Table 10-3. Note the name of the disorder, etiology (causing factor), signs and symptoms, and treatment and method of prevention (if any).

TABLE 10-3   Disorders of the Integumentary System

DISORDER	ETIOLOGY	SIGNS AND SYMPTOMS	TREATMENT AND PREVENTION
			Antibiotics and isolation to prevent infection
	Increased section of oil due to increased hormone secretion		
		Three forms: lesions; spot or growth that does not heal; or a mole that changes color, size, thickness, or texture	
		Skin blisters, itches, cracking, especially between the toes	
	Prolonged pressure and hypoxia to affected tissues		
		Itching of the scalp, white flakes	
	Virus	Papule, plantar warts may disappear	

Applying Your Knowledge

1. The hereditary condition that results in a shortage of melanocytes in the skin is called _____. One of the problems that may result from this condition is damage to the vision because _____ _____ _____ _____.

2. One fungal condition of the skin that may occur in people using the same gym area is called _____ _____.

3. A preventable sore of the skin and underlying tissues resulting from pressure is called _____ _____.

4. A very contagious bacterial infection of the skin that is common in children is called _____.

5. The three forms of skin cancer are _____, _____, and _____. The most serious form is _____. A fourth form, Kaposi's sarcoma, has become associated with the infection commonly called _____.

Applying Standard and Transmission-Based Isolation Precautions

The Communicable Disease Center has established special procedures, such as wearing gloves, masks, and gowns, to prevent the spread of infection. The procedures used depend on the method by which the pathogen is spread. In 1987, universal body substance isolation precautions were developed and recommended for use with all clients. These precautions require that the health care worker provide barriers between the blood and body fluids of the client and all others. Chapter 3 in the textbook provides further information regarding universal precautions.

Guidelines for control of bloodborne pathogens were developed to control the spread of hepatitis.

Examining the Evidence

1. Who in the health care setting has the responsibility of following universal precautions?

   _____

   _____

   _____

2. Describe how an undiagnosed infection could have been spread throughout the health care facility before universal precautions?

   _____

   _____

   _____

3. Hepatitis A is a virus spread by the fecal-oral route. Describe a chain of events that might take this bacterium from a client in one room to a client in another room.

   _____

   _____

   _____

4. What are some measures used by public health care providers and community leaders to prevent the spread of hepatitis A?

   _____

   _____

   _____

Sun Protection

Use the Internet to investigate the activity of the sun and UV rays.

Suggested Link

EPA: http://www.epa.gov/sunwise/uvindex.html

Questions

1. What is the UV index?

_____

_____

_____

2. What factors affect the UV index?

_____

_____

_____

3. What is the forecast in your area today? What sun protection measures are suggested for that rating?

_____

_____

_____

Topics of Interest

Use the Internet to investigate and write an essay on one of the following topics of interest relating to skin.

Morgollon's (unexplained dermopathy)

Suggested Link

CDC: http://www.cdc.gov/unexplaineddermopathy/investigation.html#how_long2%23how_long2

Seasonal Affective Disorder (SAD)

Suggested Link

Skin Cancer Org: http://www.skincancer.org/sad-article-2009.html

Tattoos

Suggested Link

Mayo Clinic: http://www.mayoclinic.com/health/tattoos-and-piercings/MC00020

Essay

Cardiovascular System

Find the key terms in the word search puzzle and define them in the spaces provided.

```
R H N R Q G N V F W M F C J S E Y K A S
Y H A D F T O E W K K E O I O L N N U T
K T Y V K Z I S Q A I X S I Y O Y J R E
E G O T E Q T S J G D O N A V T J U L T
V X P T H T A E R X N F I R I S C J A H
D B C M Z M L L P E A W R O M A V N G O
B N K A W R U L T R H P Q O O I J W H S
D K O V R Y C S C C M K M Z T D D S C C
Z Y I I D D R T R X X G R T V C L T A O
S Y S T E M I C C I R C U L A T I O N P
E P M V B O C O Z M Y N B G E A Y O O E
N D J G N W Y S V X F R P C J B S X S D
I R R P C K R Y U E T C A R T N O C X X
N X H S N Y A L Y C R R Y N P S E P G K
N K N T N B N I N V H S B D O Q Z C C Y
Y O S Y S T O L E L R O I L A R U C Q L
P P S T L C M M X P T E Y O L Q O O A U
I P X N E B L T O O R Z Y K N H N C F F
N G A W I R U F D G Y S G M X B Q M V Z
B R V J A Q P Y K C C J U D S W Q X Q L
```

1. Cardioversion:_____

2. Contract: _____

3. Coronary: _____

4. Diastole:_____

5. Infarction: _____

6. Pulmonary circulation: _____

7. Rate:_____

Continued

109

8. Rhythm: _____

9. Stenosis: _____

10. Stethoscope: _____

11. Systemic circulation: _____

12. Systole: _____

13. Vessel: _____

ABBREVIATIONS

Match each of the following abbreviations with the phrase that best describes its meaning or function. Then write the phrase or name for each of the abbreviations in the spaces provided.

Abbreviation	Meaning or Function
1. _____ CAD	a. "Bad" cholesterol
2. _____ CHF	b. "Good" cholesterol
3. _____ ECHO	c. Area of the heart that starts a contraction
4. _____ HDL	d. Disease of the arteries that supply blood to the legs and arms
5. _____ ICD	e. Disease of the vessels that supply blood to the heart
6. _____ LDL	f. Images created using ultrasonic waves
7. _____ OPTN	g. Inability of the heart to pump enough blood through the body
8. _____ PAD	h. Internal heart defibrillator
9. _____ SA	i. Organization that monitors and manages transplants
10. _____ SPECT	j. Process that takes photos and makes a 3D computerized image

1. CAD: _____

2. CHF: _____

3. ECHO: _____

4. HDL: _____

5. ICD: _____

6. LDL: _____

7. OPTN: _____

8. PAD: _____

9. SA: _____

10. SPECT: _____

1. The structures of the cardiovascular system are the _ _ _ _ _ and the _ _ O _ _

 _ _ _ _ _ _ _.

2. _ _ _ O _ _ _ circulation refers to the path of the blood from the intestines, gallbladder, pancreas, stomach, and spleen through the liver.

3. The heart has four chambers, called _ _ O _ _ and _ _ _ _ _ _ _ _ _ _ _.

4. Three main types of blood vessels are _ _ _ _ _ _ _ _, veins, and

 _ _ _ _ _ _ _ _ _ _ _.

5. There are _ _ _ _ _ body locations where the pulse can be counted.

6. Blood _ _ _ _ _ O _ _ is the force of the blood against the walls of the

 _ _ _ _ _ _ _ _.

7. The "lub-dup" sound of the heart results from the opening and closing of the _ _ _ _ _ _.

8. The pattern of electrical activity in heart contractions can be measured graphically with an

 _ O _ _ _ _ _ _ _ _ _ _ _ _ _ _ _ _.

9. Three cardiovascular system disorders that may be treated with a change in diet are atherosclerosis,

 _ _ _ _ _ _ _ _ _ _ _ _ _ O, and O _ _ _ _ _ _ _ _ _ _

 _ _ _ _ _ _ _ _ _ _.

10. Cardiac arrhythmia is a disturbance of the heart's _ _ O _ _ _ caused by a defect in the heart's O _ _ _ _ _ _ _ cells or by damage to heart tissue.

Use the circled letters to form the answer to this jumble. Clue: What is the circulation called when it travels from the heart to the lungs and back?

 _ _ _ _ _ _ _ _ _

Identifying Structures of the Heart

Use Figure 11-2 in the textbook to label the diagram of the heart in Figure 11-1. Shade the heart with red (oxygenated) and blue (deoxygenated) to indicate the oxygen content of the blood in the heart. In the spaces provided in Table 11-1, trace the path of the blood through the body and indicate whether the blood in each of the structures is oxygenated or deoxygenated. Indicate where the blood will go when it leaves each structure listed.

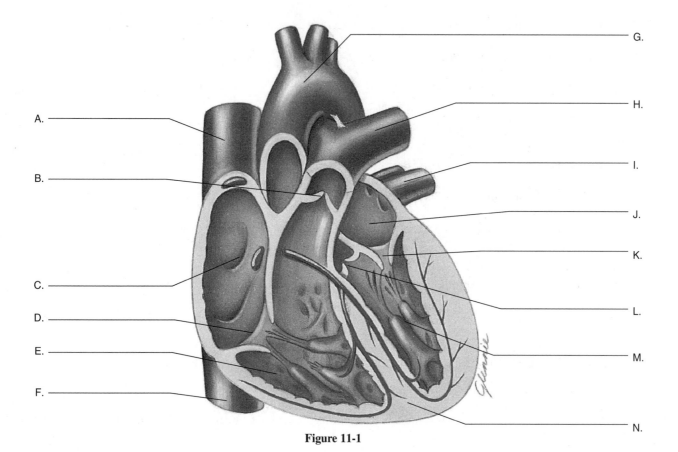

Figure 11-1

TABLE 11-1   Heart Structure

STRUCTURE	OXYGENATED OR DEOXYGENATED	BLOOD GOES FROM HERE TO THE...
Body	Both	
Lungs	Both	

Identifying Blood Vessels

Use Figure 11-4 in the textbook to label the blood vessels in Figure 11-2. Shade the portion of the diagram that contains deoxygenated blood.

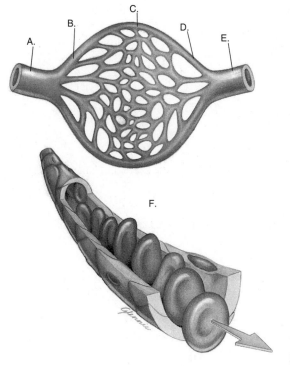

A. _____

B. _____

C. _____

D. _____

E. _____

F. _____

Figure 11-2

Identifying Principal Arteries and Veins

Use Figure 11-5 in the textbook to label the principal arteries and veins in Figure 11-3. Indicate the eight arteries commonly used to measure a pulse rate with an asterisk (*).

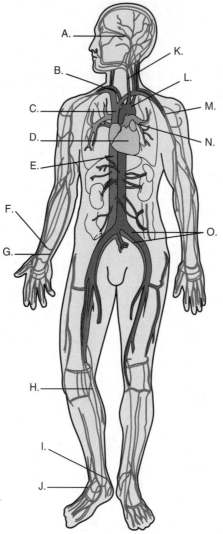

Figure 11-3

A. _____   F. _____   K. _____

B. _____   G. _____   L. _____

C. _____   H. _____   M. _____

D. _____   I. _____   N. _____

E. _____   J. _____   O. _____

Identifying Disorders of the Cardiovascular System

Complete the table of cardiovascular disorders in Table 11-2 using information provided in Chapter 11 of the textbook. Note the name of the disorder, etiology (causing factor), signs and symptoms, and treatment and method of prevention (if any).

TABLE 11-2   Disorders of the Cardiovascular System

DISORDER	ETIOLOGY	SIGNS AND SYMPTOMS	TREATMENT AND PREVENTION
	Defect in heart's pacemaker or damage to heart tissue		
	Bacterial infection that begins in the throat		
		Vessels lose elasticity, resulting in shortness of breath or fainting due to a shortage of blood supply	
			Treatment may include surgery to clear blocked coronary arteries or drugs to dissolve clots
	May be congenital	Abnormal blood flow may sometimes be heard over area of weakness in blood vessel	
	Prolonged sitting or standing		Surgical removal of clotted veins or dissolving drugs
		Veins enlarged and ineffective, leading to swelling bluish veins, redness, and pain	

Applying Your Knowledge

1. The disorder that results in damage to the heart muscle is called _____.

2. One of the complications that may result from _____ is the development of an embolus.

3. In some cases, the sound of abnormal blood flow may be heard in the condition called an _____.

4. The condition that results in more than 50% of the deaths in the United States each year is called _____.

5. The condition that commonly occurs in people who stand for long periods is called _____.

Interpreting Electrocardiographs

Using the ECG pattern in Figure 11-4, answer the following questions regarding the tracing.

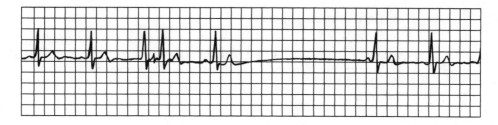

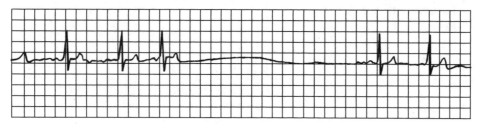

Figure 11-4

Examining the Evidence

1. What kind of heart activity does this ECG pattern represent?

_____

_____

_____

2. Why would or would not this condition be life threatening?

_____

_____

_____

3. What is the objective of treatment for a person with this ECG pattern?

_____

_____

_____

4. Why are ECG studies often performed with the person exercising, such as in a treadmill study?

_____

_____

_____

116

5. Why would it be necessary to perform a continuous ECG study using a portable monitor with a log of activities? Give at least two reasons.

_____

_____

_____

Calculating Heart Rates

The ECG pattern can also be used to calculate the heart rate. The tracing is made on grid paper that progresses at a standard recording rate of 25 mm/sec. Figure 11-5 illustrates the time required to record in each of the boxes of the ECG grid paper. To determine the rate, count the number of small boxes and multiply by 0.04 seconds.

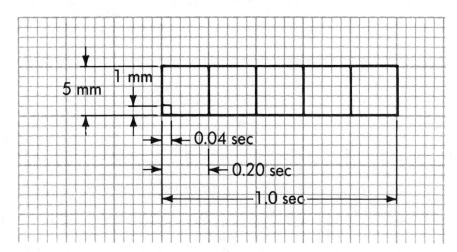

Figure 11-5

Calculate the heart rate for each of the illustrated ECG patterns in Figure 11-6, A and B.

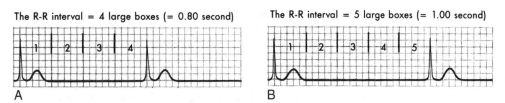

Figure 11-6

Calculate the time interval between each of the heartbeats in the ECG pattern in Figure 11-7.

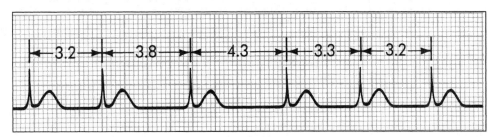

Figure 11-7

Examining the Evidence

1. The rate of the heart described in Figure 11-6, A, is _____ beats/min.

2. The rate of the heart described in Figure 11-6, B, is _____ beats/min.

3. If the heart is regular, the rate can be determined by dividing 300 by the number of large boxes in the R-R interval. Why is this true?

   _____

   _____

   _____

4. By how many seconds would you multiply the R-R interval measurement if you counted the boxes that are 5 mm instead of the smallest boxes, which are 1 mm in length?

   _____

   _____

   _____

5. Draw an ECG that shows a rate of 100 beats/min on the grid paper in Figure 11-8.

Figure 11-8

INTERNET ACTIVITIES

Heart Health Quizzes

Use the following link to complete at least three of the online heart quizzes. Write a description of your results for each.

American Heart Organization: http://www.americanheart.org/presenter.jhtml?identifier=3039196

QUIZ NAME	DESCRIPTION OF RESULTS

Mysterious Heart

Use the Internet to watch the video *PBS Mysterious Heart*. Write a paragraph or essay to describe the story of one of the three patients described.

PBS: http://www.pbs.org/wnet/heart/episode3/index.html

12 Circulatory System

VAPID VOCABULARY

Find the key terms in the word search puzzle and define them in the spaces provided.

```
Q S U N X Z M U R E S U K P K J Y
Y E A H O M A M D X N N M D D R A
D T U V Y I T I Q S E R Y L T Y B
O Y S B K T T G S G U F T E N O M
B C I Y X H P A R A T Z M E Q I K
I O T M S B E L K L O X S N J D
T B N K C F L I D U T P X F P R E
N M J Y G L E F P O G I L A B X T
A O M D A P V B H S V A E A Q Z Y
Q R G L N H I P K H M T O L Y D C
J H U G R G O A M M Y R Y C T B O
Y T R H P R I M A C C M S I I M R
R E I E T M K T O L B N J A N U H
Z G A C E P I K D X Y I N W U F T
G R E N A O U N P F P P M B M X Y
C P A M N E I O D T O C C M M A R
S M J O L V Y D M J P G L L I Z E
```

1. Allergen: _____

2. Anemia: _____

3. Antibody: _____

4. Coagulation: _____

5. Erythrocyte: _____

6. Immunity: _____

7. Inflammation: _____

8. Leukocyte: _____

9. Plasma: _____

Continued

10. Serum: _____

11. Spectrophotometry: _____

12. Thrombocyte: _____

ABBREVIATIONS

Match each of the following abbreviations with the phrase that best describes its meaning or function. Then write the phrase or name for each of the abbreviations in the spaces provided.

Abbreviation	Meaning or Function
1. _____ CBC	a. Carries oxygen and carbon dioxide in red blood cells
2. _____ DVT	b. Clotting that usually occurs in legs
3. _____ HA	c. Condition caused by a virus that does not always have symptoms
4. _____ Hct	d. Contains at least six tests to study blood
5. _____ HCV	e. Fights disease and infection
6. _____ Hgb	f. Genetic disorder that causes problems with blood clotting
7. _____ PT	g. Lives 90-120 days only
8. _____ RBC	h. Measures the amount of time it takes for blood to clot
9. _____ TIBC	i. Measures the amount of iron in the blood
10. _____ WBC	j. Measures the amount of RBCs in the blood

1. CBC: _____

2. DVT: _____

3. HA: _____

4. Hct: _____

5. HCV: _____

6. Hgb: _____

7. PT: _____

8. RBC: _____

9. TIBC: _____

10. WBC: _____

JUST THE FACTS

1. _ _ _ Ⓞ _ _ _ _ _ _ is the study of blood.

2. Erythrocytes contain a protein called _ _ _ _ _ Ⓞ _ _ _ Ⓞ, which carries oxygen to all cells and removes carbon dioxide.

3. _ _ _ _ _ Ⓞ _ _ _ _ _ fight disease and infection.

4. Platelets, also called _ _ _ _ _ _ _ Ⓞ _ _ _ _ _, promote clotting to prevent blood loss.

5. Type AB blood is called the _ _ _ Ⓞ _ Ⓞ _ _ _ recipient because it has no _ Ⓞ _ _ _ _ _ _ _ _ in the plasma to react with other blood cells.

6. Lymph has two important functions, which are maintenance of the _ _ ◯ _' _ fluid

   _ _ _ _ _ _ _ ◯ and providing immunity.

7. Three disorders of the circulatory system that are forms of cancer are Hodgkin's disease,

   _ _ _ _ _ _ _ _ _, and _ _ _ _ _ _ _ _ _ ◯ _ _ _ _.

8. Two disorders of the circulatory system that are genetic are _ _ _ _ _ _ _ _ _ ◯ _ and sickle

   cell _ _ _ _ _ _.

9. _ ◯ _ _ _ _ _ _ _ _ transfusion is the collection and transfusion of a person's own blood.

10. _ _ _ _ _ _ _ _ _ ◯ may be donated through a process called *apheresis*.

   Use the circled letters to form the answer to this jumble. Clue: What is the person who can donate blood to all people called?

   _ _ _ _ _ _ _ _ _ _   _ _ _ _ _

CONCEPT APPLICATIONS

Identifying Hematocrit Values

Use Figure 12-1 in the textbook to color and label the diagram of a hematocrit in Figure 12-1. In the spaces provided in Table 12-1, describe the components of each part.

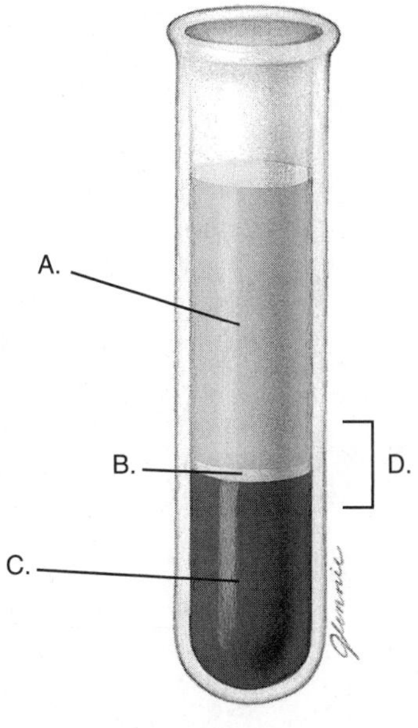

A.

B.

C.

D.

A. _____

B. _____

C. _____

D. _____

Figure 12-1

TABLE 12-1   Blood Components

BLOOD PART	COMPONENTS
Plasma	
Formed elements	

Identifying Formed Elements of Blood

Use Table 12-1 in the textbook to label the diagram of the formed elements of the blood in Figure 12-2. In the spaces provided in Table 12-2, describe the main function of each part.

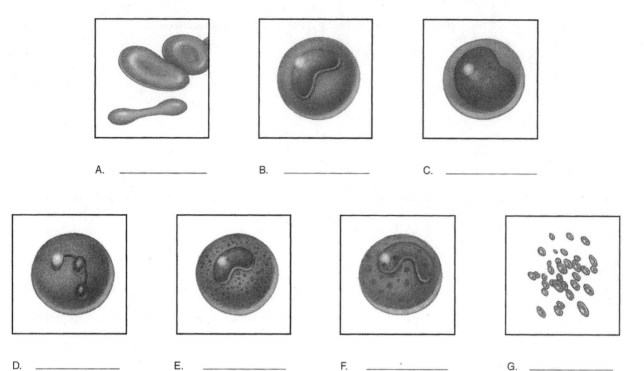

A. _____ B. _____ C. _____

D. _____ E. _____ F. _____ G. _____

Figure 12-2

TABLE 12-2   Formed Elements

ELEMENT	MAIN FUNCTION
A.	
B.	
C.	
D.	
E.	
F.	
G.	

Determining Blood Compatibility

Table 12-3 shows the antigens (agglutinogens) found on the red blood cells (RBCs) of the major blood groupings. The plasma of each of the blood groups contains antibodies that react and clot if incompatible antigens are present.

TABLE 12-3   Blood Antigens and Antibodies

BLOOD TYPE	ANTIGENS ON RBCs	ANTIBODIES IN PLASMA
A	A	Anti-B*
B	B	Anti-A†
AB	A and B	None
O	none	Anti-A and Anti-B

*Causes blood to clot if B antigen is present.
†Causes blood to clot if A antigen is present.

The compatibility of blood types can be easily demonstrated using colored water or pencils. Complete the following activity using color pencils.

Draw a container and color it blue to represent a Type B Blood recipient. "Add" Type O Blood (clear) and the color remains blue. They are compatible. Color the container red to represent a Type A donor and the color changes to purple. The blood would clot. They are not compatible.

Repeat the activity by "pouring" a donor color into a recipient color to determine which blood types are compatible. Use the information to complete Table 12-4, indicating safe transfusion possibilities.

TABLE 12-4   Blood Compatibility

BLOOD TYPE	CAN DONATE BLOOD TO:	CAN RECEIVE BLOOD FROM:
A		
B		
AB		
O		

Questions

1. Which blood type is the "universal donor"? _____

2. Which blood type is the "universal recipient"? _____

Identifying Disorders of the Circulatory System

Use the textbook to provide the missing information about circulatory disorders in Table 12-5. Note the name of the disorder, etiology (causing factor), signs and symptoms, and treatment and method of prevention (if any).

TABLE 12-5   Disorders of the Circulatory System

DISORDER	ETIOLOGY	SIGNS AND SYMPTOMS	TREATMENT AND PREVENTION
	Sex-linked genetic defect of blood coagulation		
		Fatigue, shortness of breath, pallor, rapid heart rate	
	Acute infection such as scarlet fever		
		Painless enlargement of lymph nodes, appears most often in men	
			Elevation of the affected part, anticoagulants, surgery
		Body's immune system turns against itself, Hashimoto's disease is one example	
	Blood cancer		

Applying Your Knowledge

1. Malformed blood cells characterize the inherited blood disorder known as _____.

2. A condition that results in an abnormal increase in the number of red blood cells is called _____.

3. Hodgkin's disease results in cancer of the _____ system and often is found in people _____ to _____ years of age.

4. Myasthenia gravis and systemic lupus are both examples of conditions considered to be _____ because the body's cells turn against themselves.

5. Bone marrow transplantation and isolation to prevent infection are just two treatments used for the condition of _____, which is often called _____.

AIDS Testing

Currently the courts are considering many cases involving individual rights pertaining to testing for diseases and drugs, particularly for HIV (the AIDS virus). In the past, many states required testing for the syphilis bacterium before a marriage license could be granted. To date, no routine testing program for HIV has been established, although several have been proposed.

Those who oppose routine testing for HIV fear that testing might lead to discrimination against infected individuals. Additionally, a positive result (indicating the presence of the virus) without adequate education and counseling might cause serious psychological problems for those tested.

Those who are in favor of testing think that more information is needed to determine how widespread the disease has become. They also believe that people who come in contact with someone carrying the virus have the right to know.

These issues and the following questions do not have a right or wrong answer. They ask for your opinion based on your personal beliefs. Discussion of these issues may help you become aware of your own feelings and beliefs.

Examining the Evidence

1. Why would you or would you not support routine testing for HIV?

_____

_____

_____

2. In what situations, if any, would you support the right of a victim of a crime, a health care worker, or an emergency rescue worker to require testing for HIV in someone with whom contact of body secretions has occurred?

_____

_____

_____

3. Do you feel that HIV and AIDS are being handled correctly by the Centers for Disease Control and Prevention and other supervising agencies? Explain your answer.

_____

_____

_____

Forensic Serology

Forensic serology is the study of body fluids to provide legal evidence. The pattern of the stain and the amount of blood may help determine the activity that occurred during a crime. The blood grouping antigens can be used to help determine to whom the blood belonged.

Examining the Evidence

1. Why can blood typing identification alone be used to exclude certain suspects but cannot be used to determine specifically a person's presence?

_____

_____

_____

2. When a suspect is accused of a crime and blood is found at the scene, explain why you think the officials should or should not have the right to ask for a blood sample.

_____

_____

_____

127

Chapter **12** **Circulatory System**

3. What are at least three criminal situations in which blood or other body secretions may be used as criminal evidence?

_____

_____

_____

INTERNET ACTIVITIES

Blood Types

Read the information about blood typing in the links that follow, and practice typing patients by completing the simulation.

Suggested Resources

Nobelprize.org—Information: http://nobelprize.org/educational_games/medicine/landsteiner/readmore.html
Blood Typing Simulation: http://nobelprize.org/educational_games/medicine/landsteiner/index.html

Questions

1. What is the blood type of the older man? What blood can be used for his transfusion?

_____

2. What is the blood type of the woman with red hair? What blood can be used for her transfusion?

_____

3. What is the blood type of the man with pink hair? What blood can be given to him?

_____

4. What happens to your patient if you give the wrong blood?

_____

_____

_____

Anemia

Anemia is the most common blood disorder. There are more than 400 types of anemia. Anemia results in the body cells not getting enough oxygen. The person experiences fatigue, shortness of breath, pallor, and rapid heart rate. Complete the information about anemia in Table 12-6.

Suggested Resources

WebMd: http://www.webmd.com/a-to-z-guides/understanding-anemia-treatment
Mayo Clinic: http://www.mayoclinic.com/health/SEARCH/Search

TABLE 12-6   Types of Anemia

ANEMIA	CAUSE	TREATMENT
Aplastic anemia		
Iron deficiency		
Pernicious		
Sickle cell		
Thalassemia		

13 Respiratory System

VAPID VOCABULARY

Find the key terms in the word search puzzle and define them in the spaces provided.

```
U P O M F A B D G C T S N J J
O U B O U R E J A A C B J S B
C L N D R N A N C A P A R K O
A M E T Y K I H P D F Q Z B U
N O X C G S Y T D S N Z G V A
O N Z X I P P N S O Y L K Q J
I A P Z N L G H I A Y D G H S
T R O E N O I T A R I P S N I
A Y A P N E A A P G W D G F A
R C I N O R H C B O I F E M E
I J K A I K I G Q N N A G M N
P N N P B R A D Y P N E A X P
S H X N Y T V Z T D L J K K U
E E R S W V F V S H Z W V W E
R E J G D D L J P V Y R C S J
```

1. Apnea: _____

2. Bradypnea: _____

3. Chronic: _____

4. Cilia: _____

5. Dysphagia: _____

6. Dyspnea: _____

7. Eupnea: _____

8. Expiration: _____

9. Inspiration: _____

10. Mediastinum: _____

11. Phlegm: _____

12. Pulmonary: _____

13. Respiration: _____

14. Tachypnea: _____

ABBREVIATIONS

Match each of the following abbreviations with the phrase that best describes its meaning or function. Then write the phrase or name for each of the abbreviations in the spaces provided.

Abbreviation	**Meaning or Function**
1. _____ ARDS	a. Amount of air in a normal breath
2. _____ CF	b. Amount of air that can be breathed in with effort
3. _____ CO	c. Amount of air that can be breathed out with effort
4. _____ COPD	d. Death of a baby from an unknown cause
5. _____ ER	e. Genetically caused
6. _____ IR	f. Group of chronic respiratory disorders
7. _____ SIDS	g. Related to automobile exhaust
8. _____ TB	h. Respiratory illness caused by a bacteria
9. _____ TV	i. Swelling of respiratory tissues after breathing in foreign substances
10. _____ VC	j. Total amount of air that can be breathed in and out with effort

1. ARDS: _____

2. CF: _____

3. CO: _____

4. COPD: _____

5. ER: _____

6. IR: _____

7. SIDS: _____

8. TB: _____

9. TV: _____

10. VC: _____

JUST THE FACTS

1. Both the _ _ _ _ _ ◯ _ _ _ and _ _ _ _ _ _ _ _ _ _ _ _ nervous systems control respiration.

2. The _ _ _ _ _ _ _ are hollow spaces in the bones of the skull that open into the nasal cavity.

3. Flaps of tissue protect the respiratory system from swallowed food or saliva. The flap that covers the nasal tract is called the _ _ _ _ _, and the one that covers the trachea is called the _ _ _ _ _ ◯ _ _ _ _.

4. Capillaries in the walls of the alveoli exchange oxygen and carbon dioxide by the process of

_ _ _ _ _ _ _ _ _.

5. The diaphragm _ _ _ _ _ _ _ _ _ and moves downward during inhalation.

6. The amount of air that can be brought into the lungs is called

_ _ _ _ _ _ _ _ _ _ _ _ ◯ _ _ _ _ _ _.

7. Chronic obstructive pulmonary disease is a group of chronic respiratory disorders that include

   _ _ _ _ _ _, chronic bronchitis, and _ _ _ _ $\bigcirc$ _ _ _ _

   _ _ _ _ _ _ _ _ _.

8. Two disorders of the respiratory system that are caused by a virus are _ _ _ _ _ _ _ _ _ _ _

   and a $\underset{\smile}{\bigcirc}$ _ _ _.

9. One respiratory system disorder that is directly linked to smoking is _ _ _ _ $\bigcirc$ _ _ _ _ _.

10. The respiratory disorder that has had an increased incidence since 1991 and is the most common fatal infectious

    disease in the world today is _ _ $\underset{\smile}{\bigcirc}$ _ _ _ _ _ _ _ _ _ _ _.

Use the circled letters to form the answer to this jumble. Clue: What substance is linked to cancer of the esophagus and ulcers?

_ _ _ _ _ _ _

CONCEPT APPLICATIONS

Identifying Structures of the Respiratory System

Use Figure 13-1 in the textbook to color and label the diagram of the respiratory system in Figure 13-1. In the spaces provided in Table 13-1, describe the function of each part.

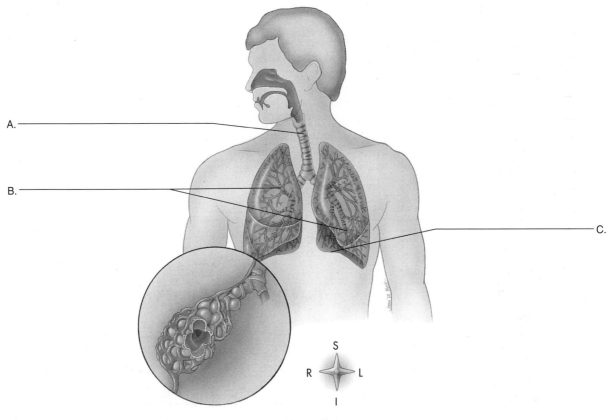

A.

B.

C.

S
R L
I

Figure 13-1

TABLE 13-1   Functions of Respiratory System Structures

SYSTEM PART	MAIN FUNCTION
Alveoli	
Bronchi and bronchioles	
Diaphragm	
Nasal cavity	
Pharynx	
Sinuses	
Tonsils and adenoids	
Trachea	

Reading a Normal Lung Volume

Use Figure 13-3 in the textbook to indicate the correct volume in liters for each of the readings in Figure 13-2. In the spaces provided in Table 13-2, describe what each of the categories represents in relation to breathing.

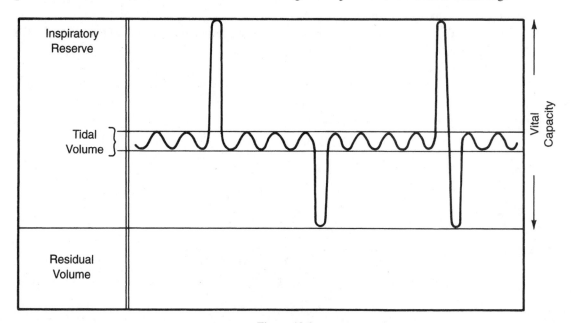

Figure 13-2

TABLE 13-2   Lung Volume Readings

LABORATORY READING	WHAT THE READING REPRESENTS
1. Residual volume	
2. Inspiratory reserve	
3. Expiratory reserve	
4. Tidal volume	
5. Vital capacity	

134

Identifying Disorders of the Respiratory System

Use the textbook to provide the missing information about the respiratory disorders in Table 13-3. Note the name of the disorder, etiology (causing factor), signs and symptoms, and treatment and method of prevention (if any).

TABLE 13-3 Disorders of the Respiratory System

DISORDER	ETIOLOGY	SIGNS AND SYMPTOMS	TREATMENT AND PREVENTION
	Caused by one or more than 200 viruses		
		Heavy cough and mucus production leaning to thickening of the bronchial walls	
	Upper respiratory infection or changes in atmospheric pressure		
	Virus, bacteria, chemical, or aspiration of fluid		
		Affects pharynx, larynx, and nose; may cause loss of voice or hoarseness	
	Bacteria transmitted through the air		
			Surgical removal of lung, chemotherapy, and radiation

Applying Your Knowledge

1. An infection that affects the nose, pharynx, or larynx is often called an _____.

2. One of the respiratory system disorders that has increased in incidence and has developed resistance to antibiotics is _____.

3. A buildup of carbon dioxide in the blood can lead to a condition called _____.

4. When air or fluid enters the space around the lungs, it is called _____.

5. A chronic condition in which the alveoli lose their elasticity is called _____.

Performing a Lung Volume Reading

The volume of air moved into and out of the lung may be used to measure the ability of the body to supply oxygen to the cells. If a wet spirometer is not available for this activity, a large, water-filled jar on which the volume is indicated may be substituted (Figure 13-3). Read all directions before beginning the activity. Laboratory activities should be performed under the supervision of a qualified professional only.

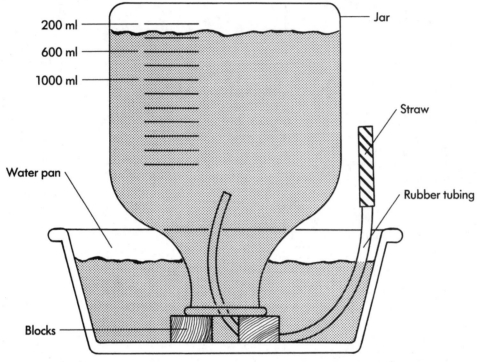

Figure 13-3

Equipment and Supplies

Disposable mouthpieces
Wet spirometer or jar apparatus

Directions

1. Work in groups of at least two people.
2. Assemble a wet spirometer for lung volume readings. Read the manufacturer's instructions before beginning. Some wet spirometers require **inspiration** of air instead of **exhalation** as later described. Exhalation is used to measure when the jar apparatus is used.
3. Place a disposable mouthpiece in the breathing tube.
4. Do not look at the gauge during breathing trials. Your partner should read all measurements.
5. To measure the tidal volume, breathe at a normal rate for several minutes. When the normal volume of air for one breath is inhaled through the mouth, gently exhale through the mouthpiece. Perform this measurement three times, and compute the average of the resulting volumes.

Trial 1 _____ liters

Trial 2 _____ liters   Average = _____ liters

Trial 3 _____ liters   Tidal Volume

6. To measure your inspiratory reserve, inhale as much air as possible. Breathe the air gently through the mouthpiece until you reach the end of a normal breath. This measurement includes the tidal volume. Perform this measurement three times, and compute the average of the resulting volumes.

Trial 1 _____ liters

Trial 2 _____ liters   Average = _____ liters

Trial 3 _____ liters   Inspiratory Reserve + Tidal Volume

Because the inspiratory reserve that you measured contains the tidal volume, you must subtract the average tidal volume from the measured inspiratory reserve to get the true value of the inspiratory reserve.

Average = _____ liters
Total Inspiratory Reserve

7. To measure expiratory reserve, breathe normally several times. After a normal breath has been exhaled, gently blow any remaining air through the mouthpiece. Perform this measurement three times, and compute the average of the resulting volumes.

Trial 1 _____ liters

Trial 2 _____ liters   Average = _____ liters

Trial 3 _____ liters   Expiratory Reserve

8. To measure vital capacity, inhale as much air as possible and gently blow through the mouthpiece. Gently exhale as much air as possible through the mouthpiece. Perform this measurement three times, and compute the average of the resulting volumes.

Trial 1 _____ liters

Trial 2 _____ liters   Average = _____ liters

Trial 3 _____ liters   Vital Capacity

9. Use a color pen or pencil to chart your results in Figure 13-4. Compare your results with the normal lung volume reading.

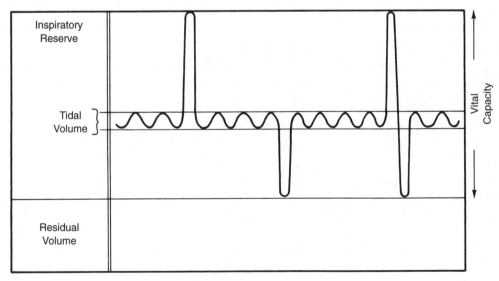

Figure 13-4

Drawing Conclusions

1. Why is the average of three volume measurements used to determine the laboratory results?

_____

_____

_____

2. What is the value of your residual volume? Why can't this value be measured?

_____

_____

_____

3. *Vital capacity*, by definition, is the sum of the inspiratory reserve, tidal volume, and expiratory reserve. Add these three values as they were measured in the laboratory activity. How does this number compare with the volume of the vital capacity that was measured in the activity? Why may these values differ?

Inspiratory Reserve + Tidal Volume + Expiratory Reserve = _____

Measured Vital Capacity = _____

_____

_____

_____

4. Would the vital capacity of an athlete be larger or smaller than that of someone who does not exercise regularly? Explain your answer.

_____

_____

_____

5. List three possible sources of error in this activity.

_____

_____

_____

Demonstrating the Effect of Smoking on Lung Tissue

Read all directions before beginning the activity. Laboratory activities should be performed under the supervision of a qualified professional only.

Equipment and Supplies

Cigarette and match or lighter
Cotton balls
Irrigation syringe or basting utensil
Microscope
Microscope slide and cover slip
Prepared microscope slide of cancerous lung tissue
Prepared microscope slide of normal lung tissue

Directions

1. Place a cigarette in the tip of an irrigation syringe that has been filled loosely with about 1 inch of cotton.
2. "Smoke" the cigarette by pulling air into and pushing it out of the syringe using the plunger. Note: It is preferable to "smoke" the cigarette outside of the classroom or under a ventilation hood.
3. Prepare a dry mount slide of the cotton after the cigarette has been "smoked."
4. Prepare a dry mount slide of cotton that has not been exposed to the cigarette.
5. Examine the slides under a microscope and compare. Sketch the cotton in the spaces provided in Figure 13-5.
6. Examine slides of normal lung tissue and cancerous tissue. Sketch the tissue in the spaces provided in Figure 13-6.

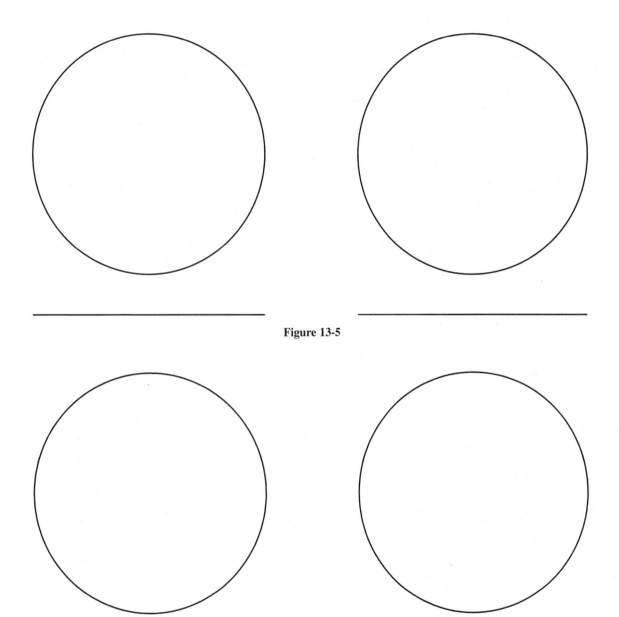

Figure 13-5

Figure 13-6

Drawing Conclusions

1. What is the residue that can be observed on the cotton after the cigarette smoke has passed through it?

2. How does the normal lung tissue compare with the cancerous tissue in appearance?

3. How might the effect of smoking on the cotton and lung tissue be compared?

4. Why would the high number of blood vessels in the lung tissues make these tissues more likely to suffer damage from cigarettes than other tissues, such as the skin?

5. If the current cost of a pack of cigarettes is $7.00, compute the cost of a pack-a-day smoker for 1 year. Assume that this amount of money is placed in an account that earns 7% interest each year. Compute the value of the money in 5 years and 10 years. (*Hint:* Remember that the amount to be calculated each year should include the interest earned from the previous year.)

CRITICAL THINKING

Smoking Choices

The rights of the nonsmoker and smoker have become a source of conflict for many people. Laws have been enacted to protect the nonsmoker from "secondhand" smoke by limiting smoking areas and requiring the availability of nonsmoking areas.

Health insurance companies offer lower rates to corporations that offer smoking cessation programs for their employees.

Examining the Evidence

1. Should the rights of nonsmokers be considered more important than those of smokers? Why or why not?

2. Do you believe that a law should be enacted to restrict or eliminate smoking entirely? Explain your answer.

_____

_____

_____

3. With more than 300,000 deaths attributed to smoking each year, why do you think that the number of smokers is actually increasing in some age groups?

_____

_____

_____

4. Most insurance companies give a discount for household policies if the occupants are nonsmokers. They do this because statistics indicate that smokers present a higher risk of fires and other related household claims. What other factors could be considered by an insurance company to determine rates?

_____

_____

_____

5. Some health insurance companies will not cover expenses because of respiratory illness in smokers. Would you support this policy? Why or why not?

_____

_____

_____

Changes in Air Pressure

The weight of the air or atmosphere around the earth is approximately 14.7 pounds per square inch ($1.03 \, kg/cm^2$). This measurement is defined as 1 atmosphere of pressure. Atmospheric pressure decreases with increased altitude and increases as a person goes under water during activities such as scuba diving.

Each 33-foot (10 m) increment of seawater depth increases the pressure 1 atmosphere. At this depth, the person is lower than 2 atmospheres of pressure (1 from the air above sea level and 1 from the pressure of the water).

The primary effect of air pressure for the diver is the volume or density of the air. In a closed container, such as a tank or lung, the volume of the air at 2 atmospheres is reduced due to the increased pressure. This inverse relationship between pressure and volume is called *Boyle's law*. As the volume of the air decreases at greater depths, the diver needs more air to fill the lungs.

Boyle's law: At a constant temperature, the volume of a gas varies inversely with the pressure exerted on it.

Examining the Evidence

1. How would the volume or density of a liter of air at the top of a mountain compare with that in the same container of air at sea level?

_____

_____

_____

2. Why might a person who does not usually live at a high altitude become short of breath when at a high altitude? What might the person do to correct this situation?

_____

_____

_____

3. Why does the scuba diver need to ascend (go from a deep water level to the water's surface) slowly?

_____

_____

_____

4. What changes occur in the volume of air in Figure 13-7, showing a closed system descent, as the container is taken from sea level to a depth of 66 feet?

_____

_____

_____

5. What changes occur in the volume of air in Figure 13-8, showing a closed system ascent, as the container is taken from a depth of 66 feet to sea level?

_____

_____

_____

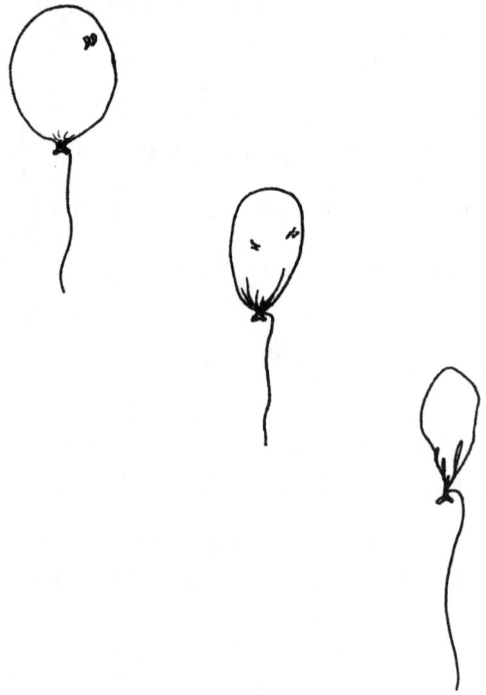

Figure 13-7

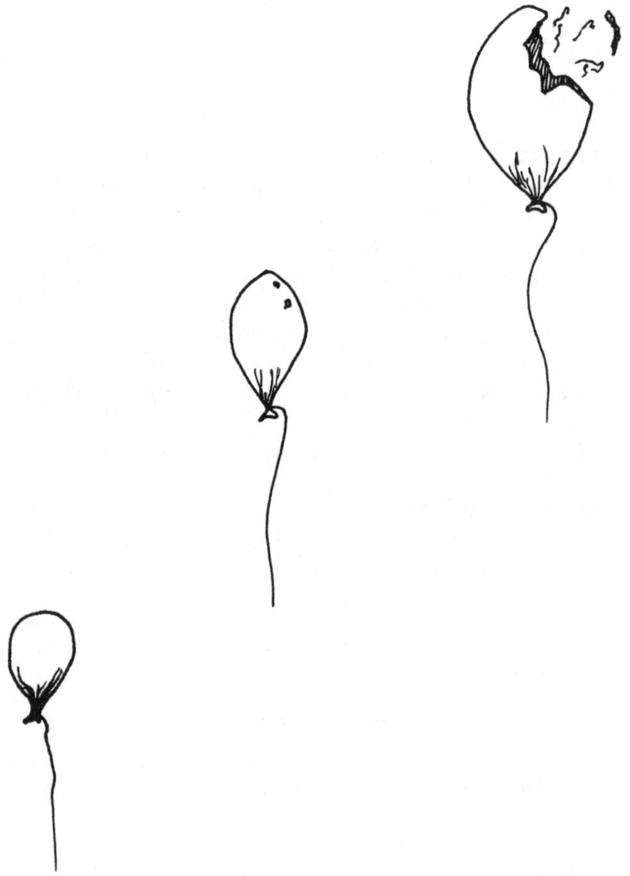

Figure 13-8

Asthma Simulation

Complete the Starlight Programs interactive activity about asthma.

Asthma Starlight Programs: http://asthma.starlightprograms.org/

Directions

1. Place the trigger items into the appropriate parts of the house and surrounding environment.
2. Complete the lung simulation.
3. Complete the peak flow meter simulation.
4. Find the "mold mob" in the house and answer the questions.

Questions

1. What are some asthma triggers?

   _____

   _____

   _____

2. What is a peak flow meter?

   _____

   _____

   _____

3. What is an asthma action plan?

   _____

   _____

   _____

4. What was your score with the "mold mob?" _____

5. Write a paragraph that compares the effects of living with asthma to living with cystic fibrosis or diabetes.

   _____

   _____

   _____

   _____

   _____

   _____

   _____

   _____

   _____

   _____

   _____

   _____

   _____

   _____

   _____

143

14 Skeletal System

Find the key terms in the word search puzzle and define them in the spaces provided.

```
A  S  E  I  T  I  M  E  R  T  X  E  D  N  M
R  W  U  L  A  I  V  O  N  Y  S  E  O  U  C
T  C  O  O  N  S  Q  Z  J  C  G  D  E  W  O
I  X  A  A  L  T  W  X  H  E  N  T  T  O  L
C  T  V  R  Z  L  E  U  N  E  S  C  L  R  L
U  U  C  B  T  L  E  E  T  O  V  I  S  R  A
L  S  Q  A  D  I  R  C  I  K  G  D  A  A  G
A  T  U  N  P  A  L  R  N  A  P  E  K  M  E
T  D  W  Q  T  M  E  A  M  A  C  P  Q  V  N
I  Q  Z  I  Z  P  O  E  G  E  C  O  S  Q  J
O  B  V  Z  I  E  N  C  J  E  K  H  I  P  C
N  E  L  O  X  T  G  T  N  T  V  T  A  J  S
X  R  E  S  O  R  P  T  I  O  N  R  G  I  A
M  F  L  B  U  R  S  A  V  A  E  O  G  K  K
U  D  T  M  I  P  M  H  D  W  V  Y  I  Y  Y
```

1. Articulation: _____

2. Bursa: _____

3. Cancellous: _____

4. Cartilage: _____

5. Collagen: _____

6. Compact: _____

7. Degenerative: _____

8. Extremities: _____

9. Ligament: _____

10. Marrow: _____

Continued

11. Orthopedic: _____

12. Periosteum: _____

13. Resorption: _____

14. Synovial: _____

15. Tendon: _____

ABBREVIATIONS

Match each of the following abbreviations with the phrase that best describes its meaning or function. Then write the phrase or name for each of the abbreviations in the spaces provided.

Abbreviation	Meaning or Function
1. _____ BMD	a. Also called degenerative joint disease
2. _____ bx	b. Any one of several tests used to determine densitometry of bones
3. _____ CT	c. Break in a bone
4. _____ CTS	d. Caused by repetitive movement of the median nerve
5. _____ DEXA	e. Pain and stiffness in joints with unknown cause
6. _____ DPA	f. Scan that compares x-rays taken at different angles
7. _____ fx	g. Scan that uses magnetic and radio waves to make images
8. _____ MRI	h. Scan that uses two energy x-rays to determine bone density
9. _____ OA	i. Scan that uses two photons to determine bone density
10. _____ RA	j. Technique that removes cells from tissue for examination

1. BMD: _____

2. bx: _____

3. CT: _____

4. CTS: _____

5. DEXA: _____

6. DPA: _____

7. fx: _____

8. MRI: _____

9. OA: _____

10. RA: _____

1. Bone tissue is composed of inorganic Ⓢ _ _ _ _, blood vessels, nerves, and

   _ _ _ _ _ _ _ _.

2. The skeletal system consists of two major groups, called the Ⓐ _ _ _ _ skeleton and the

   _ _ _ _ _ _ Ⓔ _ _ _ _ _ skeleton.

3. Bones are classified by _ _ _ _ _ as long, short, flat, or irregular.

4. The sinus cavities make the skull lighter and the voice sound _ Ⓞ _ _ _ _ _ _.

5. The _ _ Ⓝ _ _ _ _ _ _ _ _ are openings in the cranium that close by the second year

   after birth.

6. Freely movable joints include hinge, _ _ _ Ⓥ _, and _ _ _ _ _ _ _ _ joints.

7. The adult has 32 teeth after the _ _ _ _ _ _ _ _ Ⓢ or primary teeth are replaced.

8. Three disorders of the skeletal system that involve an abnormal curvature of the spine

   include _ _ _ _ _ _ _ _ _, _ _ Ⓞ _ _ _ _ _, and

   _ _ _ Ⓢ _ _ _ _ _.

9. Two disorders of the skeletal system that involve the teeth include dental _ _ _ _ Ⓔ _ and

   _ Ⓔ _ _ _ _ _ _ _ _ _ _ _.

10. A common disorder of the skeletal system that is a repetitive stress injury is _ _ Ⓞ _ _ _

    _ _ _ _ _ _ _ _ _ _ _ _ _ Ⓔ _.

   Use the circled letters to form the answer to this jumble. Clue: What is one of the functions of the skeletal system?

   _ _ _ _ _ _ _ _ _ _ _ _ _

Identifying Skeletal Bones

Use Figure 14-1, A and B, in the textbook to label the diagrams of the anterior and posterior skeletal system in Figure 14-1, A and B. Use two colors to indicate the axial and appendicular skeleton in each.

Anterior

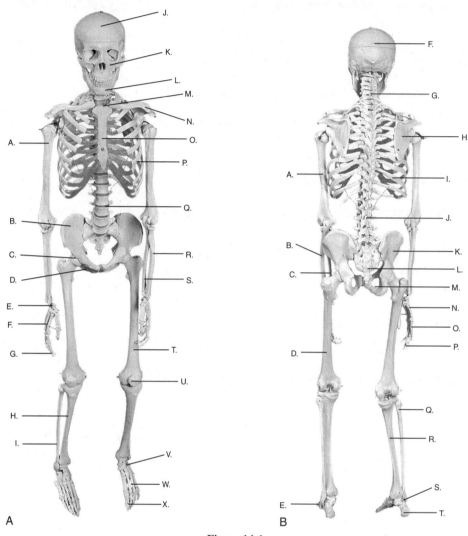

Figure 14-1

A. _____   I. _____   Q. _____

B. _____   J. _____   R. _____

C. _____   K. _____   S. _____

D. _____   L. _____   T. _____

E. _____   M. _____   U. _____

F. _____   N. _____   V. _____

G. _____   O. _____   W. _____

H. _____   P. _____   X. _____

Posterior

A. _____   I. _____   Q. _____

B. _____   J. _____   R. _____

C. _____   K. _____   S. _____

D. _____   L. _____   T. _____

E. _____   M. _____

F. _____   N. _____

G. _____   O. _____

H. _____   P. _____

Identifying Cranial Bones

Use Figure 14-2 in the textbook to label the diagram of the cranial structures in Figure 14-2.

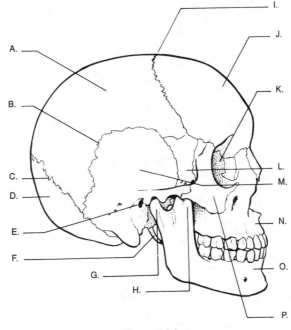

Figure 14-2

A. _____   G. _____   M. _____

B. _____   H. _____   N. _____

C. _____   I. _____   O. _____

D. _____   J. _____   P. _____

E. _____   K. _____

F. _____   L. _____

Identifying Teeth

Use Figure 14-4 in the textbook to label the teeth of the mouth in Figure 14-3.

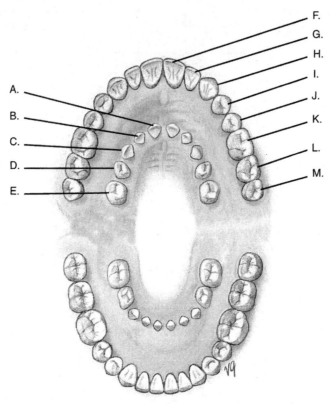

Figure 14-3

A. _____

B. _____

C. _____

D. _____

E. _____

F. _____

G. _____

H. _____

I. _____

J. _____

K. _____

L. _____

M. _____

Identifying Structures of the Long Bone

Use Figure 14-8 in the textbook to label the structures of the long bone in Figure 14-4.

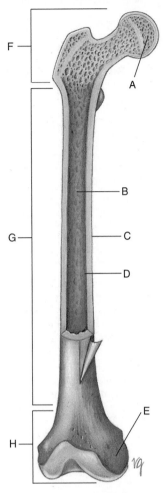

Figure 14-4

A. _____

B. _____

C. _____

D. _____

E. _____

F. _____

G. _____

H. _____

Identifying Disorders of the Skeletal System

Use the textbook to provide the missing information about skeletal system disorders in Table 14-1. Note the name of the disorder, etiology (causing factor), signs and symptoms, and treatment and method of prevention (if any).

TABLE 14-1 Disorders of the Skeletal System

DISORDER	ETIOLOGY	SIGNS AND SYMPTOMS	TREATMENT AND PREVENTION
			Pain medication, bed rest, possible surgical correction
		Abnormal lateral curvature of spine	
	Gout, trauma, infection, may be unknown		
		Inflammation of tissues around teeth; bleeding and tender gums	
		Numbness, tingling, burning sensation in hand	
	Weakening of bones, especially in women after menopause		
	Congenital	May cause paralysis and nervous system disorders because of pressure on spinal nerves	

Applying Your Knowledge

1. A group of disorders (usually of unknown cause) that result in stiffness of the joints is collectively called

_____.

2. Pressure from repetitive movements of the wrist may lead to a condition called _____.

The symptoms of this condition may include _____ and _____.

3. _____ is a condition in which the thoracic spine curves abnormally, whereas

_____ is a condition in which the lumbar spine is malformed. Of these two conditions,

the one that may cause lower back pain is _____.

4. The condition that results when bones move out of their normal location but that does not include a fracture is called _____.

5. Affecting 90% of adults, the condition that causes most tooth loss in adults is called

_____.

INVESTIGATIONS

Cast Application

Plaster casts are applied to the body to immobilize, support, and protect an injured area during healing. They also may be used to prevent or correct bone deformities. Casts are fitted or molded above, around, and below the affected area to provide traction. The material used for casting is usually plaster of Paris or calcium sulfate diphosphate. To make this material, gypsum is reduced to powder by removing the water. The powder can be placed in gauze for easy application. When water is added to the gauze, the plaster hardens and dries in any form.

The bandages for casting are made in varied widths and have "setting" speeds ranging from 2 to 18 minutes to become solid. After the cast sets into a solid form, the process of drying completely takes approximately 10 to 15 minutes longer. The strength of the cast and the drying time are determined by the number of layers of gauze applied. Usually five to seven layers are used. The formation of crystals of plaster produces heat during the drying process. A newly set cast is called *green*.

The person wearing a cast should be instructed in its proper care to ensure good results from the application. Proper care includes skin care, elevation, isometric exercises, and observation. The area of exposed skin should be washed and dried regularly. Application of lotion on the exposed area will help prevent excess drying of the skin. Massaging the exposed skin will increase circulation and promote comfort. The skin should be inspected regularly to detect any injury, such as bruising or damaged skin. A mirror may be used for this purpose if the area is difficult to see.

The skin area under the edge of the cast should be wiped regularly with a washcloth soaked in rubbing alcohol and wrapped around a finger to reduce the sensation of itching. This area under the cast should not be scratched, and foreign objects should not be inserted into the cast. Broken skin under the cast may become infected.

Whenever possible, the area of casting should be elevated to reduce swelling. If a pillow is used to elevate the area, the cast should be secured with a towel pinned to the pillow to prevent accidental slipping. Correct body alignment should be considered at all times to promote comfort and prevent problems resulting from impaired circulation.

Isometric exercises may be used during the time the cast is worn to prevent loss of muscle strength. During exercise, the joint or broken bone should not be moved.

The following are observations that may indicate that a problem has occurred with the casted area. When these conditions occur, the person should be instructed to seek medical attention.

- Reduced capillary refill (speed of blood return to toenails or fingernails)
- A musty smell
- An increase in body temperature
- A warm or hot spot on the skin around the casting area
- A tingling sensation
- Numbness
- Swelling
- Coldness of the skin
- Pale or cyanotic (bluish) skin
- Paralysis
- Drainage from the casting area

Nausea, vomiting, abdominal pain, and distention may indicate cast syndrome with a full body cast.

Read all directions before beginning the activity. For the following activity, disposable gloves may be worn, if preferred, when applying a cast because the plaster may stick to the hands. Laboratory activities should be performed under the supervision of a qualified professional only. To prevent accidental injury, casting is practiced on a mannequin.

Equipment and Supplies

Alcohol
Bucket of warm water
Gloves
Knife
Mannequin
Plastic wrap
Soap
Stockinette

Directions

1. Prepare the skin around the area of cast application by cleaning it with soap and water. Alcohol may be used to dry the skin thoroughly. Some physicians also apply talcum powders to prepare the skin.
2. Place a soft knit material or stockinette over the area to be casted.
3. Sheet wadding or padding may be applied over the stockinette. The sheet wadding and stockinette are applied smoothly to prevent skin breakdown from wrinkling. Liquid adhesive may also be used.
4. Line two buckets and the table surface to be used with plastic. The plaster material will bind permanently to many surfaces. Plaster waste is never disposed of in sinks because it will solidify in the pipes.
5. Place lukewarm water in the buckets. The temperature of the water determines how fast the plaster sets. Warmer water speeds the setting time and also produces more heat during drying.
6. Grasp the plaster roll by placing your thumb in the middle of the roll.
7. Submerge the roll of plaster vertically (on end) in the water.
8. When bubbles stop rising from the roll, grasp both ends of the bandage to prevent unraveling and remove it from the water.
9. Squeeze the bandage slightly to remove water by forming a bulge in the center of the roll. Do not twist or wring the bandage. Plaster bandages are applied when still sopping wet.
10. The part to be casted must be kept in the correct alignment, or position, throughout the procedure. After the procedure, the area may be radiographed to confirm correct alignment.
11. Wrap the plaster bandage around the area from the most distal end toward the heart. Apply each roll so that it covers half of the width of the previous roll. Bandages are applied directly over the stockinette, fitting closely but not tightly enough to hinder circulation in the area. Bandages may be soaked two at a time for quicker application. If bandages soak in the water too long, some of the plaster material may be lost.
12. Smooth the edges and surface of the cast by rubbing the cast with an open hand in a continuous motion during application.
13. Trim the plaster with a knife as necessary to smooth edges or to provide windows for circulation and observation of tissues.
14. Casts may be split on both sides (bivalve) to relieve pressure from swelling if needed. Remove excess plaster from the skin with a sponge dampened with a solution of vinegar and water.
15. Place the cast in an elevated position after it has cooled. During drying, the cast should be exposed to the air to allow the release of the heat produced. Be sure to handle the wet cast gently; this prevents indentations from fingers that might cause pressure sores.
16. Observe the cast for evidence of drying, approximately 15 to 20 minutes. Table 14-2 presents characteristics of wet and dry casts.

TABLE 14-2   Characteristics of Wet and Dry Casts

WET CAST	DRY CAST
Musty smell	Odorless
Dull sound when tapped	Hollow sound when tapped
Gray and lustreless	White and shiny
Cool to touch	Room temperature

Drawing Conclusions

1. What might the presence of numbness, tingling, or paralysis in a limb with a cast indicate?

_____

_____

_____

2. What might the presence of pale or cyanotic skin indicate?

_____

_____

_____

3. What might drainage from the casting area indicate?

_____

_____

_____

4. Why is a stockinette used for skin preparation?

_____

_____

_____

CRITICAL THINKING

Rheumatoid Conditions

The term *rheumatoid* refers to the tissues around the joints. Rheumatoid conditions are chronic, disabling, and usually incurable. They include rheumatoid arthritis, systemic lupus erythematosus, progressive systemic sclerosis, Lyme disease, and myositis, as well as many types of arthritis. More than 60 million Americans have a form of rheumatic disease.

Edema resulting from rheumatoid conditions may be managed with aspirin or aspirin-like NSAIDs (nonsteroidal anti-inflammatory drugs). Pain relievers and exercise programs help the person retain use of the affected joints. In some cases, corticosteroids may be administered, and surgery may be performed to correct resulting deformities. In some specific cases, antimalarial drugs, gold salts, penicillamine, sulfasalazine, and immunosuppressive agents may be used to control symptoms. Diet also may have a positive effect. People with rheumatoid conditions have been the victims of many types of quackery.

Examining the Evidence

1. Why do you think people with rheumatoid conditions would be candidates for a quackery cure or treatment?

_____

_____

_____

2. Some victims of the AIDS virus develop arthritis. In what way do you think this disease may be related to the rheumatoid conditions?

_____

_____

_____

3. Management of rheumatoid conditions is expensive because of the necessary medications and treatments. What are two methods by which the costs may be reduced?

_____

_____

_____

Chapter **14** **Skeletal System**

INTERNET ACTIVITIES

Interactive Body

Use the following Internet link to practice placement of bones in the Interactive Body.

Suggested Link

BBC Science Interactive Body:
http://www.bbc.co.uk/science/humanbody/body/interactives/3djigsaw_02/index.shtml?skeleton

Questions

1. What was your score?

_____

Mouth Power

Use the following Internet link to complete each of the six modules of MouthPower Online. Make a list of important tips from each module.

University of Maryland MouthPower.org: http://www.mouthpower.org/mouthpower.cfm

MouthPower Module Tips

1. Food Station— _____

_____

_____

2. Tobacco Station— _____

_____

_____

3. Cleaning Station— _____

_____

_____

4. Your Tooth Story— _____

_____

_____

5. Dental Time Warp— _____

_____

_____

6. Creativity Corner— _____

_____

_____

15 Muscular System

Find the key terms in the word search puzzle and define them in the spaces provided.

```
I  M  S  K  C  J  J  R  E  X  W  J  Z  R  D
A  O  O  U  P  A  R  A  L  Y  S  I  S  E  V
T  T  N  R  N  P  U  N  U  P  R  F  S  V  C
T  S  R  U  J  O  D  G  Y  X  H  V  R  O  S
S  X  I  O  L  A  T  E  L  E  K  S  N  M  A
X  Y  Q  N  P  F  C  O  E  S  Y  T  S  E  R
Z  Y  J  F  O  H  O  F  G  H  R  M  U  M  C
P  E  X  Y  U  G  Y  M  P  A  H  Y  L  I  O
Y  Z  M  B  E  S  A  O  C  F  G  A  U  R  M
E  R  U  T  C  A  R  T  N  O  C  L  M  P  E
M  I  Y  M  D  T  I  I  N  T  P  G  I  Z  R
E  R  U  T  S  O  P  O  I  A  L  I  T  H  E
A  K  W  Y  N  F  A  N  C  V  K  A  S  K  I
K  G  D  I  O  X  K  V  I  S  C  E  R  A  L
Y  M  C  G  R  U  R  A  Z  H  F  S  E  C  Z
```

1. Antagonist: _____

2. Atrophy: _____

3. Contraction: _____

4. Contracture: _____

5. Dystrophy: _____

6. Myalgia: _____

7. Paralysis: _____

8. Posture: _____

9. Prime Mover: _____

Continued

157

10. Range of Motion: _____

11. Sarcomere: _____

12. Skeletal: _____

13. Stimulus: _____

14. Tonus: _____

15. Visceral: _____

ABBREVIATIONS

Match each of the following abbreviations with the phrase that best describes its meaning or function. Then write the phrase or name for each of the abbreviations in the spaces provided.

Abbreviation	Meaning or Function
1. _____ ACSM	a. Agency that gathers statistics
2. _____ ADP	b. Amount of possible movement
3. _____ ATP	c. Calculation based on weight and height
4. _____ BMI	d. Method to calculate risk of falling in older people
5. _____ CDC	e. Muscle wasting due to genetic inheritance
6. _____ DMD	f. Muscle weakness with an unknown cause
7. _____ GARS	g. Organization with treatment of sports injuries as main emphasis
8. _____ MG	h. Part of the energy cycle with two phosphates only
9. _____ PRP	i. Part of the energy cycle with three phosphates
10. _____ ROM	j. Use of blood to treat sports injuries

1. ACSM: _____

2. ADP: _____

3. ATP: _____

4. BMI: _____

5. CDC: _____

6. DMD: _____

7. GARS: _____

8. MG: _____

9. PRP: _____

10. ROM: _____

JUST THE FACTS

1. Muscle contraction is the ◯ _ _ _ _ _ _ _ of muscles when stimulated.

2. _ _ _ _ ◯ is the muscle's ability to maintain slight, continuous contraction.

3. Skeletal muscle tissue looks striated, or ◯ _ _ _ _ _, under the microscope.

4. The three parts of the skeletal muscle are the _ _ _ _ _ _, _ _ _ _ _ _ _ _ _ _ _, and ◯ _ _ _ _ _ _.

5. _ _ _ _ ◯ _ _ _ muscle lines various hollow organs, makes up the walls of blood vessels, and is found in the tubes of the digestive system.

6. Cardiac muscle is found only in the heart and is ◯ _ _ _ _ _ _ _ _ _ _ _ _ striated.

7. _ ◯ _ _ _ _ _ _ _ _ _ _ is a condition in which muscles remain contracted as a joint loses flexibility and ligaments and tendons shorten.

8. Two muscular system disorders that are caused by bacteria are _ _ ◯ _ _ _ _ _ and
_ _ _ _ _ _ _ _.

9. A muscular system disorder that includes a genetic cause in one form is _ _ _ ◯ _ _ _ _
_ _ _ _ _ _ _ ◯ _.

10. When a person chooses a sports club, some factors that should be considered include the credentials of the
_ _ _ _ _, _ _ _ _ of the facility, _ _ _ _ _ _ ◯ _ _ _ _, and ◯ _ _ _ _ _ _ _ terms.

Use the circled letters to form the answer to this jumble. Clue: What is the type of sports medicine that studies the body in motion?

_ _ _ _ _ _ _ _ _ _ _ _ _

Identifying Anterior Muscles

Use Figure 15-2A in the textbook to label the diagram of the anterior muscles in Figure 15-1.

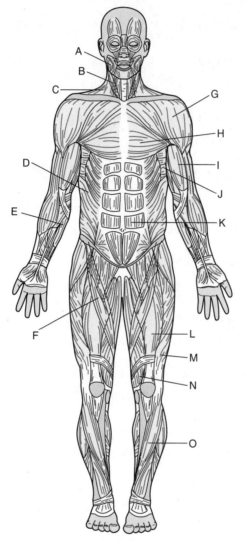

Figure 15-1

A. _____

B. _____

C. _____

D. _____

E. _____

F. _____

G. _____

H. _____

I. _____

J. _____

K. _____

L. _____

M. _____

N. _____

O. _____

Identifying Posterior Muscles

Use Figure 15-2B in the textbook to label the diagram of the anterior muscles in Figure 15-2.

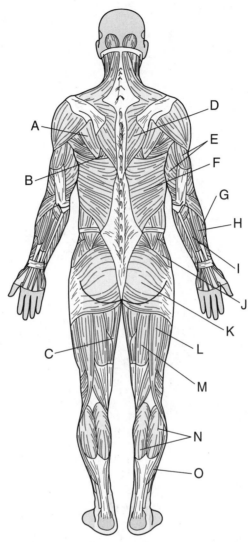

Figure 15-2

A. _____   F. _____   K. _____

B. _____   G. _____   L. _____

C. _____   H. _____   M. _____

D. _____   I. _____   N. _____

E. _____   J. _____   O. _____

Identifying Parts of the Muscle

Use Figure 15-4 in the textbook to identify the parts of the muscle in Figure 15-3. Color the muscles, bones, ligaments, and tendons different colors for identification.

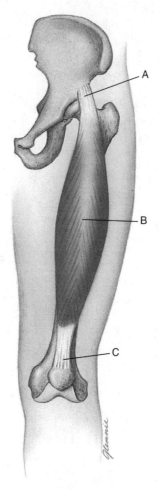

Figure 15-3

A. _____

B. _____

C. _____

Identifying Muscle Tissue Types

Use Figures 15-3, 15-7, and 15-8 in the textbook to identify the diagrams of muscle tissue types in Figure 15-4, A to C. Then label each tissue type in the spaces provided in Table 15-1. Indicate whether each of the muscle types is controlled by voluntary or involuntary action.

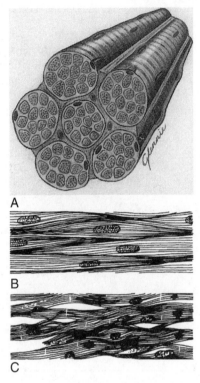

A

B

C

Figure 15-4

TABLE 15-1   Identifying Muscle Tissue Types

TISSUE TYPE	TYPE OF ACTION (VOLUNTARY OR INVOLUNTARY)
A.	
B.	
C.	

Identifying Disorders of the Muscular System

Use the textbook to provide the missing information about muscular system disorders in Table 15-2. Note the name of the disorder, etiology (causing factor), signs and symptoms, and treatment and method of prevention (if any).

TABLE 15-2   Disorders of the Muscular System

DISORDER	ETIOLOGY	SIGNS AND SYMPTOMS	TREATMENT AND PREVENTION
	Genetic		
			Bracing, surgical procedure to restore proper position and medication
		Joint loses flexibility, tendons may shorten	
			Treatment includes preventing complications; may be prevented with vaccination
	Viral infection		
	Clostridium bacteria		
	Cause unknown, considered to be autoimmune		

Applying Your Knowledge

1. Loss of flexibility in a joint, resulting in shortening of the tendons and ligaments, is called a _____ and may be caused by _____.

2. Painless, gradual atrophy of the muscles may be caused by a genetic condition called _____.

3. Often occurring in the groin area, the condition called a _____ may be treated with surgery.

4. Paralysis caused by _____ may be prevented by vaccination.

5. Caused by *Clostridium* bacteria, _____ may lead to the death of muscle tissue.

Observing Muscle Tissue

Read all directions before beginning the activity. Laboratory activities should be performed under the supervision of a qualified professional only. Care must be taken when handling chemicals and glassware. Gloves are worn when handling raw meat products.

Equipment and Supplies

Disposable gloves
Dissecting needle
Eyedropper
Forceps
Methylene blue stain
Microscope
Microscope slides and cover slips
Prepared slide of muscle tissue types
Raw pork chop or beef

Directions

1. Examine a prepared slide of each of the three muscle types under low and high power.

2. Draw each of the three muscle types as observed under high power in the spaces provided in Figure 15-5. Label the nucleus, cytoplasm, cell membrane, and striations that can be identified.

3. In a drop of water on a clean slide, tease apart a small piece of raw meat. Separate the fibers with a dissecting needle.

4. Transfer a few strands of the meat fiber to a slide that has been prepared with a dry film of dilute methylene blue stain.

5. Add a drop of water and a cover slip to the slide. Wrap the slide and cover slip in a paper towel, and gently press with your thumb or a pencil eraser to spread the fibers.

6. Observe the slide under low and then high power. Draw the specimen as observed under high power in the space provided in Figure 15-6.

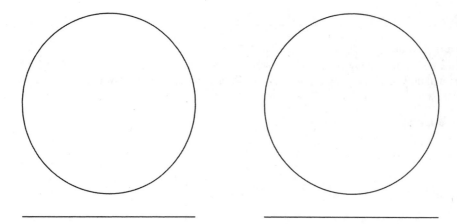

_____   _____

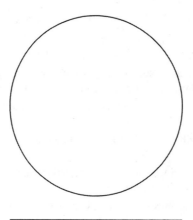

_____

Figure 15-5

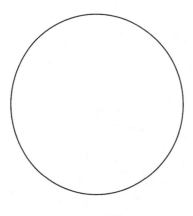

_____

Figure 15-6

Drawing Conclusions

1. Which of the prepared muscle slides looks most like the slide you made?

_____

_____

_____

2. Which of the prepared muscle tissue slides is the most easily identified by microscopic examination? Explain why this is so.

_____

_____

_____

3. Based on the observation of the slide you prepared, what do you think happens to the muscle tissue in a muscle tear injury?

_____

_____

_____

Observing Muscle Movement

Read all directions before beginning the activity. Laboratory activities should be performed under the supervision of a qualified professional only. Care must be taken when handling chemicals and glassware. Gloves are worn when handling raw meat products.

Equipment and Supplies

Raw chicken wing
Disposable gloves
Dissecting tray
Forceps
Paper towels
Scissors

Directions

1. Rinse a complete raw chicken wing under running water. Dry it with paper towels, and place it in a dissecting tray.
2. Pull the skin away from the muscle with forceps, and cut the skin the length of the wing. Take care to avoid cutting the underlying muscle tissue. Observe the thin connective tissue (mesentery) between the skin and the muscle tissues.
3. With a probe, separate the skin from the muscle. If the skin over the joints is difficult to remove, a scalpel may be used in this area. It is not necessary to remove the skin from the wing tip.
4. Rinse and dry the chicken wing after removing the skin. Observe and diagram the chicken wing in the space provided in Figure 15-7.
5. Observe the tendons at the end of the muscles. Notice the shape of the muscles.
6. Grasp the wing at the shoulder and tip. Pull the wing to extend the length and bend it back to its original shape. Observe how the muscles contract during movement. Identify the muscles that work in pairs.
7. Observe the largest muscle of the wing to determine its origin and insertion.
8. Draw the chicken wing as it appears after removal of the skin. Label the muscle origin, insertion, body, tendons, and bones in Figure 15-8. Use arrows to indicate the direction of the antagonistic muscles in the diagram.
9. Dispose of the chicken wing and gloves in the appropriate container. Clean the laboratory equipment and return it to the designated area as instructed.
10. Wash your hands thoroughly with soap and water.

Chapter **15** **Muscular System**

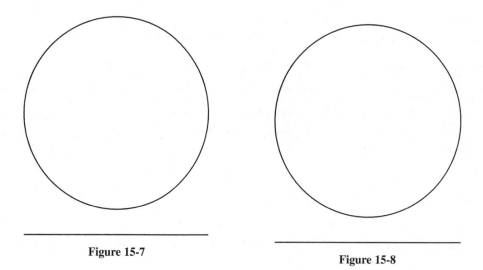

_____

Figure 15-7

_____

Figure 15-8

Drawing Conclusions

1. Use Figure 15-5 in the textbook to name two antagonistic, or opposing, muscles in the human body.

_____

_____

_____

2. Why are disposable gloves worn when handling raw meat?

_____

_____

_____

Demonstrating Reflex Actions

Read all directions before beginning the activity. Muscles contract when they are stimulated, manipulated, or pulled by gravity. They also contract when the tendons attaching the muscles are stretched. This activity provides methods of assessing the function of the tendon reflexes. Laboratory activities should be performed under the supervision of a qualified professional only.

Equipment and Supplies

Percussion hammer

Directions

1. Arm reflexes that can be demonstrated include the biceps, triceps, and brachioradialis reflexes. To assess these reflexes, place your thumb over the tendon to hold the limb being observed.

2. Strike your thumb with a percussion hammer so that the blow is transmitted to the tendon. The percussion hammer is held between the thumb and index finger during assessment. Reflexes of both sides of the body should be tested and compared for equality. Table 15-3 indicates the location struck by the percussion hammer and the response expected for these reflexes.

3. Assess the lower limb in a similar manner. Table 15-3 also provides information about the lower limb reflexes and expected responses.

4. Record the results of the activity in Table 15-4. Use a plus sign (+) to indicate a reaction and a minus sign (−) to indicate no response.

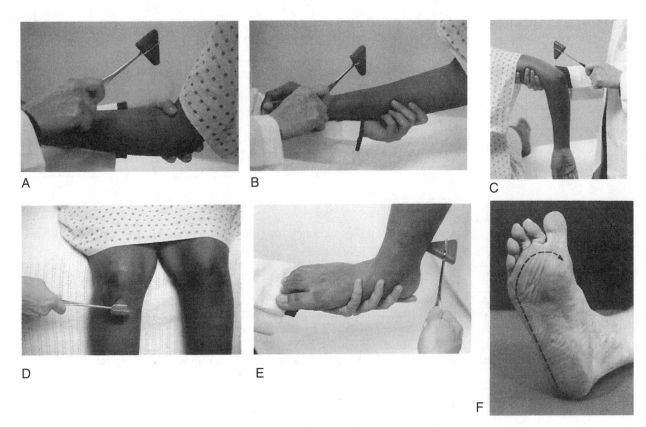

Figure 15-9

TABLE 15-3 Reflex Assessment

DISORDER	LOCATION OF THUMB	EXPECTED RESPONSE
Biceps	The arm is flexed at the elbow with the examiner's thumb over the biceps tendon in the antecubital area (Figure 15-9, A).	Flexion of the arm at the elbow
Triceps	The arm is flexed at the elbow with the examiner's thumb over the triceps tendon on the outer aspect of the arm (Figure 15-9, B).	Straightening or extension of the arm
Brachioradialis	The examiner's thumb supports the extended arm in a relaxed position while the styloid process (bony prominence on the wrist) is struck with the hammer (Figure 15-9, C).	Flexion of the arm at the elbow
Patellar	With the legs dangling free over the side of a chair or bed, tap directly below, or inferior to, the patella (Figure 15-9, D).	Extension of the leg
Achilles tendon	The foot is held in slight dorsiflexed position (Figure 15-9, E).	Plantar flexion of the foot
Plantar	Use a key, a pin, or the end of the reflex hammer to press a line from the lateral border of the sole, starting at the heel and continuing up to and across the ball of the foot (Figure 15-9, F).	Flexion of all of the toes

TABLE 15-4   Reflex Results

REFLEX	RIGHT SIDE RESPONSE	LEFT SIDE RESPONSE
Biceps		
Triceps		
Brachioradialis		
Patellar		
Achilles tendon		
Plantar		

Drawing Conclusions

1. Which of the reflexes tested showed a positive response?

_____

_____

_____

2. Which of the reflexes showed a negative response? Hypothesize why these responses were absent.

_____

_____

_____

3. List three factors that might influence the results of this activity.

_____

_____

_____

CRITICAL THINKING

Weight Training

Body building by using weights or weight training became popular with the increased interest in health and fitness. It is estimated that more than 7 million Americans exercise regularly with weights. Equipment and exercise routines have been developed to improve the strength and muscle tone in all areas of the body. After only 6 weeks of training, the benefits of weight training can be seen in the development of firmer and stronger muscles.

A high-protein diet promotes muscle mass.

Lifting weights causes the proteins that form muscle tissue to pull apart. The muscle tissue is broken down and then replaced with new tissue. The new tissue has bigger and stronger fibers than those that were destroyed. The body requires about 48 hours to regenerate the proteins of muscle tissues. For that reason, it is not a good idea to exercise the same muscle groups every day.

Weight training is an anaerobic exercise, which means it does not consume oxygen. It uses energy that is stored in the muscles. Some exercise equipment is designed for continuous use to increase the cardiovascular or aerobic benefit from lifting weights. However, combining aerobic movement and stretching with lifting weights provides an all-around fitness program.

Weights may be used in either free form or as part of a machine. Free weights, barbells, and dumbbells are not as expensive as the machinery designed for weight training. The correct equipment should be selected for the results desired.

Precautions, such as the use of correct body mechanics and stretching exercises, must be taken to prevent injury during use of all types of weights. All weight-training programs should begin slowly to prevent torn or damaged muscles and tendons.

Examining the Evidence

1. Why is the addition of stretching exercises and aerobic activity to weight training a complete program of fitness?

_____

_____

_____

2. If a person desires to lift weights every day, how could a program be designed to prevent muscle injury?

_____

_____

_____

3. What precautions are taken to prevent muscle tears when a person is lifting weights?

_____

_____

_____

INTERNET ACTIVITIES

Interactive Body

Use the following Internet link to practice placement of muscles in the Interactive Body.

Suggested Link

BBC Science Interactive Body:
http://www.bbc.co.uk/science/humanbody/body/interactives/3djigsaw_02/index.shtml?muscles

Questions

1. What was your score? _____

Physical Activity At-a-Glance

Use the information from the CDC Physical Activity and Health Report to design a program of activity for a week. Use Table 15-5 to track your progress.
Physical Activity and Health Report: http://www.cdc.gov/NCCDPHP/sgr/ataglan.htm

TABLE 15-5   Activities

ACTIVITY	DAY/TIME	CALORIES USED

Questions

1. In what other physical activities do you participate?

   _____

   _____

   _____

2. What are two of the benefits of regular physical activity that are important to you?

   _____

   _____

   _____

16 Digestive System

Digestive System

VAPID VOCABULARY

Find the key terms in the word search puzzle and define them in the spaces provided.

```
R F I L T Q O C Y F H N D B P
W T N P S N H X M Q O Y E O B
S U G W E Y D M O I P A F L T
X H E M M R V K T O Q F E U A
E C S E K T I I C V L B C S I
C X T G L F T S E A Y C A M S
I R I D A U O A T H S S T I A
D L O A L D I U S A V H I Y T
N W N G N M L P Y J L Q O X C
U B E E I E I B C V C S N N A
A D A L N D E M E S I S I T L
J D U C R R X V L L N L O S A
A B E A M E N E O F I M L S W
A D R E T C N I H P S B U U S
Q D N M A S T I C A T I O N S
```

1. Alactasia: _____

2. Bile: _____

3. Bolus: _____

4. Bulimia: _____

5. Cholecystectomy: _____

6. Chyme: _____

7. Defecation: _____

8. Deglutition: _____

Continued

173

9. Emesis: _____

10. Endoscopy: _____

11. Enema: _____

12. Flatulence: _____

13. Ingestion: _____

14. Jaundice: _____

15. Mastication: _____

16. Peristalsis: _____

17. Sphincter: _____

18. Villus: _____

ABBREVIATIONS

Match each of the following abbreviations with the phrase that best describes its meaning or function. Then write the phrase or name for each of the abbreviations in the spaces provided.

Abbreviation	Meaning or Function
1. _____ BE	a. Agency that monitors health of animals
2. _____ CDC	b. Agency that monitors the number of food poisoning outbreaks
3. _____ FDA	c. Condition that includes Crohn disease and colitis
4. _____ GB	d. Condition that leads to esophagitis
5. _____ GERD	e. Congenital narrowing of the intestines
6. _____ HAV	f. Contrast medium used to see internal organs
7. _____ HBV	g. Organ that stores bile
8. _____ IBD	h. Treatable condition with genetic cause
9. _____ PKU	i. Virus that is transmitted by contact of body fluids
10. _____ PS	j. Virus that is transmitted from feces to mouth

1. BE: _____

2. CDC: _____

3. FDA: _____

4. GB: _____

5. GERD: _____

6. HAV: _____

7. HBV: _____

8. IBD: _____

9. PKU: _____

10. PS: _____

JUST THE FACTS

1. The main function of the digestive system is to _ _ _ Ⓞ _ _ _ _ _ _ food to a form that can be used by Ⓞ _ _ _ _ _ _ _ _ _.

2. Three _ _ Ⓞ _ _ _ _ _ glands secrete an enzyme (amylase) that begins the chemical portion of the digestive process in the _ Ⓞ _ _ _.

3. In the stomach, the food _ _ _ Ⓞ _ mixes with hydrochloric acid and the enzymes pepsin and gastrin to become _ _ _ _ _.

4. Most absorption of digestive products occurs in the _ _ _ _ _ _ _ _ Ⓞ _ _ _ _ _ _ _.

5. Most of the water from ingested food is absorbed back into the blood through the walls of the _ Ⓞ _ _ _ _ _ _ _ _ _ _ _ _ _ _.

6. The digestive system has three accessory organs, which aid the process of food breakdown. They are the _ _ Ⓞ _ _ _ _ _ _, _ _ _ _ _ _ _ _ _ _ _ _ _, and _ Ⓞ _ _ _.

7. The liver has many important functions, including storage of _ _ _ _ _ _ _ and _ _ _ _ _ Ⓞ _ _, breakdown of _ _ _ _ _ _, and reprocessing of _ _ _ Ⓞ _ _ _ _ _ _Ⓞ_ _ _.

8. Two digestive system disorders that involve problems with elimination are Ⓞ _ _ _ _ _ _ _ _ and _ _ _ _ _ _ _ _ _ _ _ _ _ _ _.

9. Two digestive system disorders that have a genetic cause are _ _ _ _ Ⓞ _ _ _ _ _ _ _ _ _ _ _ and _ _ _-Ⓞ _ _ _ _ _.

10. Two digestive system disorders that are caused by a virus are _ _ _ _ _ _ _ Ⓞ _ and the Ⓞ _ _ _ _.

Use the circled letters to form the answer to this jumble. Clue: What are two of the most common eating disorders called?

_ _ _ _ _ _ _ _   _ _ _   _ _ _ _ _ _ _

Identifying Structures and Functions of the Digestive System

Use Figure 16-1 in the textbook to label and color the diagram of the digestive system in Figure 16-1. Color the accessory organs the same color. In the spaces provided in Table 16-1, describe the function of each part.

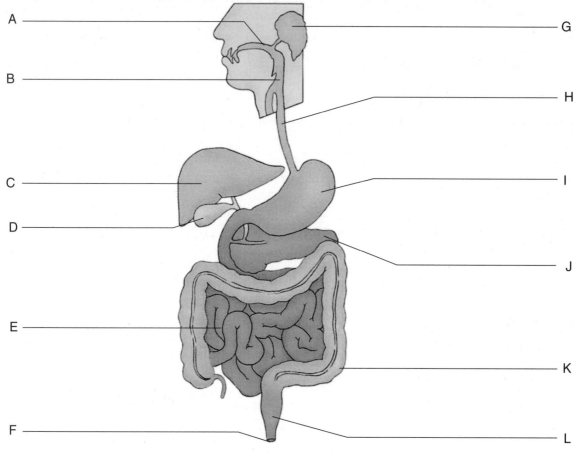

Figure 16-1

TABLE 16-1   Structures of the Digestive System

ORGAN	FUNCTION
A. Mouth	
B. Pharynx	
C. Liver	
D. Gallbladder	
E. Small intestine	
F. Anus	
G. Salivary glands	
H. Esophagus	
I. Stomach	
J. Pancreas	
K. Large intestine	
L. Rectum	

Identifying Disorders of the Digestive System

Use the textbook to provide the missing information about digestive system disorders in Table 16-2. Note the name of the disorder, etiology (causing factor), signs and symptoms, and treatment and method of prevention (if any).

TABLE 16-2   Disorders of the Digestive System

DISORDER	ETIOLOGY	SIGNS AND SYMPTOMS	TREATMENT AND PREVENTION
	Virus, transmitted in food, water, or body secretions		
	Salmonella and other bacteria		
			Emotion and stress may trigger symptoms; diet changes, medication, surgery
	Bacteria or stress		
		Flatulence, cramps, diarrhea when dairy products are ingested	
		Jaundice, skin lesions, demineralization of bones, enlargement of the liver, anemia, bleeding disorders	
			Surgical removal of the appendix

Applying Your Knowledge

1. A very common disorder of the digestive system prevents many people from enjoying milk products, such as ice cream. This condition is due to the lack of an enzyme called _____.

2. When radiographs of the intestinal tract are taken, a substance called _____ may be swallowed. It helps show the structures as it passes through the digestive tract.

3. The procedure that may be used to view the inside of the stomach or to remove gastric contents is called _____.

4. A viral infection that may result from eating contaminated food and that causes jaundice affects the _____. This condition is called _____.

5. An open sore anywhere along the digestive tract is called an _____; it may be caused by _____ that eats the lining of the stomach.

177

Dissection of a Perch

Read all of the directions before beginning this activity. Disposable gloves are worn while handling specimens that have been prepared or stored in caustic fluids. The directions are for dissection of a preserved perch. Pigeons, fetal pigs, and frogs may be used as well.

Equipment and Supplies

Disposable gloves
Preserved specimen (perch)
Dissecting tray
Forceps
Dissection scissors

Directions

1. Place the specimen for dissection on a dissecting tray.
2. Examine the teeth of the specimen, taking care to avoid cutting yourself on the sharp edges. Observe the mouth cavity.
3. Using forceps and a pair of scissors, open the abdominal cavity of the specimen carefully to avoid cutting the organs.
4. Observe the membrane surrounding the abdominal organs. Carefully loosen this membrane and move it to the side.
5. Locate the esophagus of the perch. The esophagus leads directly into the saclike stomach pouch. Observe the shape and size of the stomach.
6. The stomach leads into the intestine. The waste of the perch leaves the body through the rectum. Trace the intestine to the rectum.
7. Locate and observe the liver of the perch. Observe that the gallbladder is attached to the liver. Observe that the stomach is attached to the intestine by a small tube or duct.
8. Label the following parts of the digestive system of the perch on the lines below the diagram in Figure 16-2.

Mouth	Stomach
Intestine	Anus
Teeth	Liver
Gallbladder	Esophagus

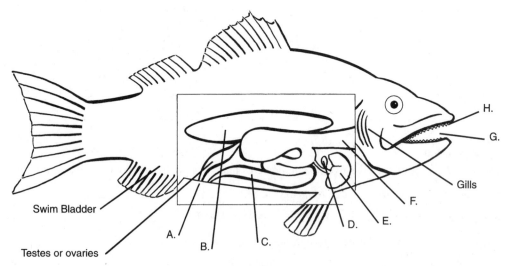

Figure 16-2

A. _____   E. _____

B. _____   F. _____

C. _____   G. _____

D. _____   H. _____

Drawing Conclusions

1. The small fish and aquatic organisms eaten by the perch are swallowed whole. What is the purpose of the teeth and mouth?

_____

_____

_____

2. The stomach of the perch is much larger than its liver. In humans, the liver is larger than the stomach. How would you explain this difference?

_____

_____

_____

3. Based on your observations of the perch's digestive system, hypothesize whether it would get more nutrition from eating frequently or less often.

_____

_____

_____

CRITICAL THINKING

Understanding Eating Disorders

Some researchers believe that the origin of eating disorders is related to a victim's need to have control of some feature of his or her life, such as appearance. By exerting control over the body, through losing weight despite hunger and signs of physical damage, the victim of the disorder feels a sense of power. Often victims believe they are fat even when they are extremely thin. The theory continues that weight loss gives the victim a sense of identity or a feeling of being competent because he or she is able to lose weight.

Authorities estimate that up to 5% of adolescent and college-age women in the United States suffer from bulimia.

Examining the Evidence

1. When eating disorders, such as anorexia nervosa and bulimia, result in obvious physical changes, such as hair loss and tooth damage, why do you think these changes do not stop the victim from purging or self-starvation?

_____

_____

_____

2. Hypothesize why the frequency of these eating disorders is increasing.

_____

_____

_____

3. Some of the signs of eating disorders include rapid weight gain or loss, preoccupation with calories, denial or defensive behavior when confronted with eating habits, unexplained vomiting, sores at the corners of the mouth, and continuous episodes of overeating without weight gain. If you observed these signs in someone you knew, what would you do?

_____

_____

_____

Harvest of Fear

Use the PBS NOVA website called Harvest of Fear to investigate genetically modified foods. Prepare a position report either for or against the use of genetically modified foods. Print and complete the video worksheet from the teachers' activity page while watching the video. Choose one of the character roles to play and complete the "Are Genetically Modified Foods Safe?" from the teachers' activity page. Hold a debate from the point of view of your role using the information gathered. If the video is not available, use the Internet to research the answers to the questions.

   PBS: http://www.pbs.org/wgbh/harvest/

   Write a paragraph to summarize your opinion about the use of genetically modified foods.

_____

_____

_____

_____

_____

_____

_____

_____

Engineer a Crop Simulation

Use the PBS Nova Harvest of Fear link to create corn larger and engineer a "supercrop."
   PBS: http://www.pbs.org/wgbh/harvest/engineer/index.html

Interactive Menu Planner

Use the National Heart Lung and Blood Institute Interactive Menu Planner to make a daily plan that meets the nutritional requirement of your personalized MyPyramid.gov plan for weight loss or gain. List the requirements of your personal plan in Table 16-3. List the meals you planned in Table 16-4.

   MyPyramid.gov Personal Plan: http://www.mypyramid.gov/mypyramid/index.aspx
   NHLBI: http://hp2010.nhlbihin.net/menuplanner/menu.cgi

TABLE 16-3   MyPyramid.gov Personal Plan

ITEM	PLAN RECOMMENDATION
Calories	
Exercise time	
Grains	
Vegetables	
Fruits	
Milk	
Meat and beans	

TABLE 16-4   Meal Selections

MEAL	ITEM	CALORIES
Breakfast (servings)		
Lunch (servings)		
Dinner (servings)		
Snack (servings)		
Total		

Questions

1. Compare your current diet plan with the one you created using the menu planner.

   _____

   _____

   _____

2. How difficult was it to create a meal that meets all of your nutritional recommendations?

   _____

   _____

   _____

17 Urinary System

VAPID VOCABULARY

Find the key terms in the word search puzzle and define them in the spaces provided.

```
C  A  I  R  U  S  O  C  Y  L  G  S  M  K  N
U  L  D  T  A  E  W  A  K  P  O  I  A  O  O
X  B  R  I  N  I  A  J  O  B  C  E  I  X  L
K  U  X  Z  U  D  R  L  X  T  M  T  R  X  I
M  M  A  S  I  R  Y  U  U  U  A  M  U  F  G
A  I  S  O  O  U  E  R  N  N  D  B  Y  A  U
I  N  V  I  R  U  I  S  I  A  U  J  P  N  R
R  U  L  I  S  T  N  R  I  Y  M  M  U  J  I
U  R  A  Y  I  Y  U  E  T  S  V  V  B  S  A
T  I  G  O  W  F  L  Q  O  X  M  A  E  G  F
A  A  N  V  T  K  D  A  A  I  R  U  S  Y  D
M  C  H  D  K  G  F  M  N  E  A  D  H  A  N
E  D  I  A  L  Y  S  I  S  I  L  B  B  R  I
H  Q  Y  Q  D  P  F  Q  V  Q  R  C  F  S  I
G  K  O  Z  Z  H  T  X  Q  Z  X  U  Y  F  O
```

1. Albuminuria: _____

2. Anuria: _____

3. Dialysis: _____

4. Diuresis: _____

5. Dysuria: _____

6. Glycosuria: _____

7. Hematuria: _____

8. Micturition: _____

9. Oliguria: _____

10. Polyuria: _____

Continued

11. Pyuria: _____

12. Urinalysis: _____

13. Urination: _____

14. Void: _____

ABBREVIATIONS

Match each of the following abbreviations with the phrase that best describes its meaning or function. Then write the phrase or name for each of the abbreviations in the spaces provided.

Abbreviation	Meaning or Function
1. _____ CAPD	a. Amount of acid or base in a solution
2. _____ ESRD	b. Condition when kidneys have lost all function
3. _____ ESWL	c. Dialysis performed in the home setting
4. _____ HD	d. Exchange of fluids using the abdominal cavity
5. _____ HPD	e. Imaging study that shows blockage in the urine system
6. _____ IVP	f. Organization that maintains the national transplant list
7. _____ KUB	g. Removal of waste products from the blood using a machine
8. _____ NKF	h. Shock wave therapy to remove kidney stones
9. _____ pH	i. Three organs of the urinary system
10. _____ UNOS	j. Voluntary group organized to prevent kidney and urinary tract diseases

1. CAPD: _____

2. ESRD: _____

3. ESWL: _____

4. HD: _____

5. HPD: _____

6. IVP: _____

7. KUB: _____

8. NKF: _____

9. pH: _____

10. UNOS: _____

1. The function of the urinary system includes regulation of the composition of _ _ _ ◯ ◯ _ _ _ _ _ and removal of _ _ ◯ _ _ _ from the blood.

2. The _ _ ◯ _ _ _ _ is the location of formation of urine and is the functional unit of the urinary system.

3. The _ _ _ _ _ _ _ _, a smooth muscular sac that expands as it fills with urine, can hold up to 1 L.

4. Urine consists of _ _ ◯ _ _ and _ _ _ _ ◯ _ _ _ _ _ _ _ _ from the breakdown of protein, hormones, electrolytes, pigments, and toxins.

5. Two disorders of the urinary system that are caused by bacteria are ◯ _ _ _ _ _ _ _ and _ _ _ _ _ _ _ _ _ ◯ _ _ _ _ _ _ _.

6. Renal calculi, commonly called *kidney stones*, are made up of _ _ _ _ _ _ _ _ and _ _ _ _ ◯ _ _ _ _ _ _.

7. Two urinary disorders that involve abnormal excretion of urine are urinary _ _ ◯ _ _ _ _ _ _ _ _ _ and urinary _ _ _ _ _ _ _ _ _.

8. Two forms of dialysis are _ _ _ _ _ ◯ _ _ _ _ _ _ and _ _ _ _ _ _ _ _ ◯ _ dialysis.

9. _ ◯ _ _ _ _ _ _ _ _ _ _ _ _ _ _ has a success rate of greater than 95%.

10. Kidney stones may be removed by _ _ _ ◯ _ _ _ or a _ _ _ _ _ _ _ ◯ _ treatment called lithotripsy.

Use the circled letters to form the answer to this jumble. Clue: What is a test of the urinary system that shows the density of the urine?

_ _ _ _ _ _ _ _ _ _ _ _ _ _ _

Identifying Structures and Functions of the Urinary System

Use Figure 17-1 in the textbook to label and color the diagram of the urinary system in Figure 17-1. In the spaces provided in Table 17-1, describe the function of each part.

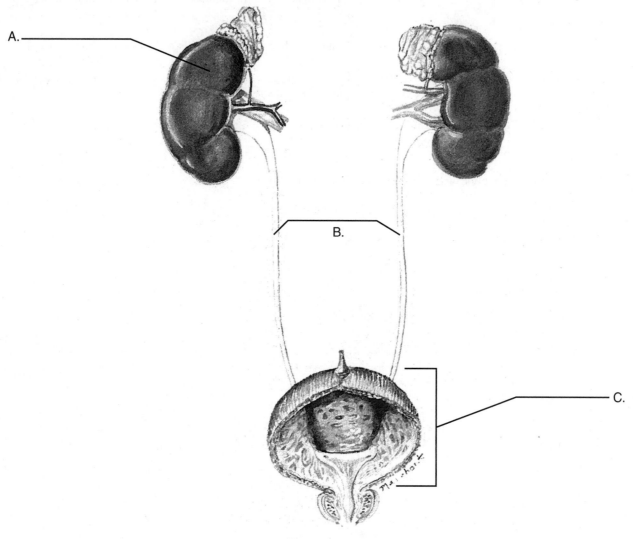

Figure 17-1

TABLE 17-1   Urinary System Structures and Functions

SYSTEM PART	MAIN FUNCTION
A.	
B.	
C.	

Identifying Structures and Functions of the Kidney

Use Figure 17-3 in the textbook to label the diagram of the kidney in Figure 17-2. In the spaces provided in Table 17-2, describe the function of each part.

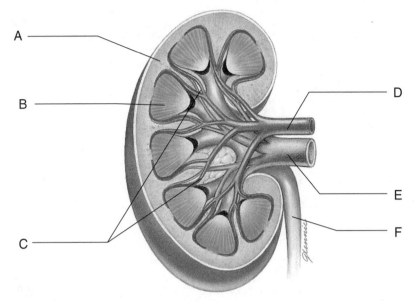

Figure 17-2

TABLE 17-2   Kidney Structures and Functions

KIDNEY PART	MAIN FUNCTION
A.	
B.	
C.	
D.	
E.	
F.	

Identifying Disorders of the Urinary System

Use the textbook to provide the missing information about urinary system disorders in Table 17-3. Note the name of the disorder, etiology (causing factor), signs and symptoms, and treatment and method of prevention (if any).

TABLE 17-3   Disorders of the Urinary System

DISORDER	ETIOLOGY	SIGNS AND SYMPTOMS	TREATMENT AND PREVENTION
		Nausea, vomiting, headache, coma	
		Swollen tissues, locally or systemic	
		Fever, lower back pain, frequent, painful, bloody urination	
	Bacteria	Painful urination, urinary frequency, blood in urine	
			Lithotripsy or surgical removal may be used
	Bacteria or chemical irritation		
	Lack of muscle control, immobility, neural damage		

Applying Your Knowledge

1. An abnormal amount of fluid accumulation in the tissues of the body is called _____.

   It may be caused by failure of the _____.

2. Another name for a kidney stone is a _____ _____. Its specific cause

   is _____.

3. Women may suffer a condition called _____ more often than men because the urethra is shorter in women than in men.

4. When the kidneys do not filter the blood, the person may experience nausea, vomiting, headache, and coma.

   Crystals may form on the skin as the body tries to rid itself of wastes in this condition, which is called

   _____   _____.

5. The treatment for kidney failure that involves removal of waste products through an artificial kidney is called

   _____.

INVESTIGATIONS

Urinalysis

Read all of the directions before beginning this activity. Urine composition may be determined through a series of simple tests. Disposable gloves are worn for handling body secretions. Laboratory activities should be completed under the supervision of a qualified professional only.

As early as AD 500, urine was studied as an indication of health.

Equipment and Supplies

Chemical "dipstick" indicator strip with reference chart
Hydrometer or graduated cylinder with urinometer
Natural or artificial urine
Paper or urine specimen cup
pH paper (or similar acid/base indicator) with reference chart

Directions

1. Collect the appropriate type of urine specimen needed for each test.

2. Observe the clarity of a fresh, routine specimen of urine. Record the appearance:

   _____

3. Note the odor of a fresh, routine specimen of urine. Describe this smell:

   _____

4. Perform a pH test using a fresh, routine specimen of urine. Litmus, Nitrazine, or hydrion paper may be used as an indicator. Each paper turns varied colors in acidic and basic solutions. Dip the bottom half of a small piece of indicator paper in the specimen. Compare the color of the paper with the chart provided with the paper. Do not touch the paper container with the urine-soaked paper while comparing the colors. Record the value of the pH of the urine:

   _____

5. Perform a specific gravity test using a fresh, routine specimen of urine. Pour the urine into a graduated cylinder or hydrometer container to a level 1 inch below the top of the cylinder. Without touching the sides of the cylinder, gently twist and release the urinometer into the urine. Read the results of the specific gravity as soon as the spinning stops. Record the value of the specific gravity:

   _____

6. Use "dipsticks" to determine the presence of any abnormal components of urine, including blood, sugar, acetone, and proteins. Follow the manufacturer's instructions for the use of each indicating stick. Record the presence of any abnormal components:

   _____

Drawing Conclusions

1. Use Table 17-2 of the textbook to determine whether the observation of clarity made in step 2 is normal. If the value is outside of the normal range, why might it be different?

   _____

   _____

   _____

2. Use Table 17-2 of the textbook to determine whether the odor noted in step 3 is normal. If the value is outside of the normal range, why might it be different?

   _____

   _____

   _____

3. In step 4, the directions state that care should be taken not to touch the pH paper container with the urine-soaked paper. Why is this important?

   _____

   _____

   _____

4. Use Table 17-2 of the textbook to determine whether the value obtained for the pH is normal. If the value is not within the normal range, why might it be different?

_____

_____

_____

5. Use Table 17-2 of the textbook to determine whether the value obtained for the specific gravity is normal. If the value is not within the normal range, why might it be different?

_____

_____

_____

6. Use Table 17-2 of the textbook to determine what the presence of any abnormal components in the urine specimen might mean, and describe the condition.

_____

_____

_____

CRITICAL THINKING

Urinary Changes with Aging

During the aging process, the kidney tissues become scarred and less efficient. Blood vessels carry blood to and from the kidneys at a lower pressure, causing less urine production. Muscle weakness in the pelvic area may lead to urine retention or inability to empty the bladder completely. In young people, urine is produced throughout the day and concentrated at night. In older individuals, the ability to concentrate urine may be lost, leading to the need to urinate during the night (nocturia). Loss of the ability to control urination is called *incontinence*. Incontinence may occur in the elderly due to infection, loss of muscle tone, or an inability to reach the toilet facilities when needed.

Examining the Evidence

1. List three methods that might be used to help an elderly person control a urinary incontinence problem.

_____

_____

_____

2. List two ways in which the problem of nocturia might be lessened.

_____

_____

_____

3. List three physical and/or psychological problems that might result from urinary incontinence or retention.

_____

_____

_____

4. How might you help a person adjust to one of the problems you identified in question 3?

_____

_____

_____

Excretion in the Body

Complete Table 17-4 by placing an "X" in the box if the waste product is removed by the part of the body listed. List other functions of the body part in the "Other Function" column. Chapter 10 of the textbook provides information about the skin. Chapter 13 of the textbook provides information about the lungs.

TABLE 17-4   Waste Products Removal

BODY PART	WASTE PRODUCT REMOVED					
	CO_2	UREA	NA^+	WATER	URINE	OTHER FUNCTION
Kidneys						
Skin						
Lungs						

Examining the Evidence

1. When a person has a failure of the kidneys, the skin may show particles of salt. Why would this be true?

   _____

   _____

   _____

2. When a person has a failure of the kidneys, the skin may appear shiny or leather-like. Why would this be true?

   _____

   _____

   _____

INTERNET ACTIVITIES

Urinary Topics

Use the Internet to research one of the following topics. Write an essay, make a poster, or make a pamphlet that describes the topic.

Enuresis
Suggested Websites
Family Doctor: http://familydoctor.org/online/famdocen/home/children/parents/toilet/366.html
Kids Health: http://kidshealth.org/kid/health_problems/bladder/enuresis.html

Cranberry Juice Remedies
Suggested Websites
Science Daily: http://www.sciencedaily.com/releases/2009/08/090824141051.htm
Medline Plus: http://www.nlm.nih.gov/medlineplus/ency/article/000521.htm

Home Dialysis
Suggested Websites
USA Today: http://www.usatoday.com/news/health/2009-08-23-dialysis_N.htm
Home Dialysis Central: http://www.homedialysis.org/learn/types/

Dialysis versus Transplant
Suggested Websites
USA Today: http://www.usatoday.com/news/health/2009-08-23-dialysis_N.htm
University of Maryland Medical Center: http://www.umm.edu/news/releases/kidcost.htm
National Kidney Foundation: http://www.kidney.org/news/newsroom/fs_new/25factsorgdon&trans.cfm

Essay

18 | Endocrine System

Find the key terms in the word search puzzle and define them in the spaces provided.

```
B L N F P E Y P E K C Y J C A E H H
N A Y I C O O T F J A Y U N I N M Y
R O S L P L L I R S N Z O F M D N P
M U L A Y O K Y S E L L B W E O F E
T P E U L S R A P I B E V Z C C F R
U O R H W M O T Y H R U P I Y R U G
N I P M X N E O O L A R P U L I O L
A D I R U S K T I D O G H H G N U Y
G W U M T F O F A S A K I U O E G C
D Z M F U G P X T B O N V A P K E E
B I S W J V N A L B O U O V Y H N M
O Z K Q I Z G X R N O L T G H U K I
N K L C P L W P O L Y D I P S I A A
S O M L A H T H P O X E E C Q C H O
T D E N O M R O H G P C C T R C R E
G P D Q J Y E C K L X N M M H A A N
E I Z A K C X L V B M Q X X Z C T R
N N R X B E K V A E E P V P M E X E
```

1. Basal metabolic rate: _____

2. Endocrine: _____

3. Exophthalmos: _____

4. Gonadotropin: _____

5. Hormone: _____

6. Hyperglycemia: _____

7. Hypoglycemia: _____

8. Immunoassay: _____

Continued

9. Polydipsia: _____

10. Polyphagia: _____

11. Polyuria: _____

12. Prostaglandin: _____

13. Puberty: _____

ABBREVIATIONS

Match each of the following abbreviations with the phrase that best describes its meaning or function. Then write the phrase or name for each of the abbreviations in the spaces provided.

Abbreviation	Meaning or Function
1. _____ ACTH	a. Also called the growth hormone
2. _____ ADH	b. Condition that can cause water intoxication
3. _____ FSH	c. Hormone produced by the placenta
4. _____ GHRH	d. Hormone that regulates growth and metabolism of the thyroid gland
5. _____ HCG	e. Pituitary hormone that can cause Cushing's syndrome if oversecreted
6. _____ ICSH	f. Pituitary hormone that regulates the amount of water excreted
7. _____ LH	g. Stimulates growth of ovaries and estrogen production
8. _____ SIAD	h. Stimulates secretion of testosterone
9. _____ STH	i. Stimulates the release of growth hormone
10. _____ TSH	j. Stimulates the release of an egg from the ovary

1. ACTH: _____

2. ADH: _____

3. FSH: _____

4. GHRH: _____

5. HCG: _____

6. ICSH: _____

7. LH: _____

8. SIAD: _____

9. STH: _____

10. TSH: _____

1. The primary function of the endocrine system is to produce (O) _ _ _ _ _ _ _ that monitor and coordinate _ (O) _ _ _ _ _ (O) _ _ _ _ _ _ _.

2. Hormones are _ _ _ _ (O) _ _ _ _ _ _ _ _ _ _ _ (O) _ secreted by the endocrine glands.

3. Three categories of hormones include _ _ _ _ _ _ hormones, _ _ _ hormones, and _ _ _ _ _ _ _ _ hormones.

4. Hormones direct body processes, including _ _ _ _ _ (O) (O) _ _ _ _ _ _ _ _ _ _, and _ _ _ _ _ (O) _ _ _ _ _ _ functions.

5. The _ (O) _ _ _ _ _ _ _ _ _ _ _ is a structure located above the pituitary gland that translates nervous system impulses into endocrine system messages.

6. The _ _ _ _ _ (O) _ _ _ gland is sometimes called the "master" gland because the hormones that it produces regulate the secretion of other glands.

7. The _ _ _ (O) _ _ _ produces hormones that regulate body metabolism.

8. The (O) _ _ _ _ _ _ _ produces the hormones that regulate transportation of sugar, fatty acids, and amino acids into the cells.

9. Insulin-dependent diabetes results when the pancreas secretes too little insulin, resulting in _ (O) _ (O) _ _ _ _ _ _ _ _ _ _ _.

10. Two disorders of the endocrine system that lead to an abnormal body size are _ _ _ _ _ _ _ _ and _ _ _ _ _ _ _ (O) _.

Use the circled letters to form the answer to this jumble. Clue: What is the disorder of the endocrine system that may lead to exophthalmos?

_ _ _ _ _ _ _ _ _ _ _ _ _ _ _

Identifying Structures and Functions of the Endocrine System

Use Figure 18-1 of the textbook to label and color the diagram of the endocrine system in Figure 18-1. In the spaces provided in Table 18-1, describe the name, function, and a hormone for each gland.

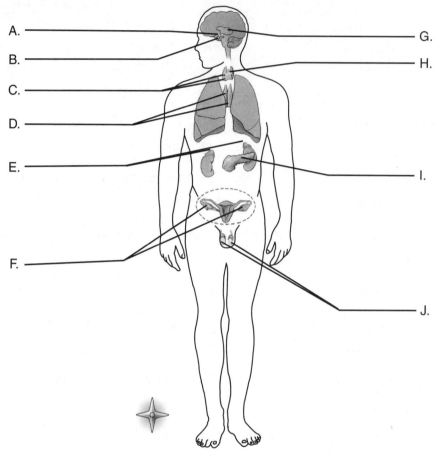

Figure 18-1

TABLE 18-1   Structures and Functions of the Endocrine System

GLAND	FUNCTION	HORMONE (EXAMPLE)
A.		
B.		
C.		
D.		
E.		
F.		
G.		
H.		
I.		
J.		

Identifying Disorders of the Endocrine System

Use the textbook to provide the missing information about endocrine system disorders in Table 18-2. Note the name of the disorder, etiology (causing factor), signs and symptoms, and treatment and method of prevention (if any).

TABLE 18-2 Disorders of the Endocrine System

DISORDER	ETIOLOGY	SIGNS AND SYMPTOMS	TREATMENT AND PREVENTION
		Normal trunk and head with shortened extremities; does not affect intelligence	
			Removal of part or all of the thyroid
			Low-carbohydrate diet with high protein
		Women may develop male sexual characteristics	
		Polydipsia, polyuria, polyphagia	
			Administration of cortisone, decrease in sodium intake, monitoring of potassium blood level
	Autoimmune disorder of iodine deficiency		

Applying Your Knowledge

1. Two hereditary conditions that are caused by different hormone imbalances and that lead to abnormal growth and appearance are _____ and _____.

2. Two conditions that result in hyposecretion of the adrenal glands are _____ and _____.

3. A person who exhibits symptoms of frequent thirst, hunger, weight loss, and increased urine output might be tested for _____.

4. Iodized salt is one method by which everyone is ensured an adequate supply of the hormone _____.

5. The test that determines the amount of energy needed by the body for functions of the resting body is called _____. A lower value in this area might indicate a problem with the _____.

Testing Urine for Sugar and Ketone

Diabetes mellitus is a disorder of the pancreas characterized by inadequate secretion of the hormone insulin. Insulin regulates the transportation of fatty acids, sugar, and amino acids into the cells. Without insulin, sugar (glucose) cannot be used as a source of energy, and fat is used instead. When fat is broken down to be used for energy, a molecule called a *ketone* is left over. Ketone is the same structure as the chemical called *acetone*. When diabetes is not controlled, the ketone and sugar molecules are carried in the blood until they are removed by the kidneys. The accuracy of the Clinitest and the Acetest is very important. The medication and food needs of the client with diabetes are based on the results of these simple tests.

Read all of the directions before beginning this activity. Disposable gloves are worn when handling body secretions, such as urine. Laboratory activities are performed under the supervision of a qualified professional only.

Equipment and Supplies

Chemical reagent strips with indicator chart
Disposable gloves
Urine specimen

Directions

1. Wear gloves when collecting and testing urine.
2. Collect a fresh, routine specimen of urine.
3. Strips treated with a special chemical reagent often are used to test for sugar and ketone in the urine. The reagent strip changes color when sugar or ketone is present in the urine. The degree of color change indicates the percentage of sugar or ketone in the specimen.
4. Hold the strip by the end that does not have the chemical squares.
5. Dip the strip in the urine.
6. Follow the manufacturer's instructions about the length of time to wait before comparing the reagent strip with the color chart on the bottle.
7. Do not touch the bottle with the urine-soaked strip.
8. Dispose of the specimen, gloves, and other supplies as directed.
9. Wash your hands thoroughly.
10. Record the results of the Clinitest for the percentage of sugar in the specimen: _____
11. Record the results of the Acetest for the percentage of ketones in the specimen: _____

Drawing Conclusions

1. Why is it important to time the exposure of the strips precisely as indicated in the instructions when checking the quantity of sugar or ketone present?

    _____

    _____

    _____

2. Why is it important to avoid touching the bottle with the urine-soaked strip?

    _____

    _____

    _____

3. What household item is generally made primarily of ketone? Why do you think it might be harmful to the body for this molecule to be present in the blood?

    _____

    _____

    _____

4. If the Clinitest and Acetest indicate the presence of sugar but no fat in the urine, what do these results mean?

_____

_____

_____

5. Blood also may be used to test for sugar levels. A small prick is made in the finger, and a drop of blood is placed on a testing strip made for this purpose. Which method would provide the most accurate reading on which to base the amount of insulin needed? Why is this true?

_____

_____

_____

6. Compare the benefits and drawbacks of using urine or blood samples for testing the sugar content of the blood.

_____

_____

_____

CRITICAL THINKING

Hormones and Adolescence

Many problems experienced by adolescents are related to hormonal changes and imbalances. For example, the age at which puberty is reached varies greatly among individuals. The development of secondary sexual characteristics at an early or late age may greatly influence the development of a positive self-concept. Diabetes mellitus is often discovered for the first time during the adolescent years. Anorexia nervosa and steroid abuse cause changes in the function of many organs, including those of the endocrine system.

Examining the Evidence

1. What do you think would be the feelings of a boy who develops secondary sexual characteristics several years later than his peers?

_____

_____

_____

2. What kind of behavior might result from this boy's feelings?

_____

_____

_____

3. What do you think would be the feelings of a girl who develops secondary sexual characteristics several years earlier than her peers?

_____

_____

_____

4. What kind of behavior might result from this girl's feelings?

_____

_____

_____

Chapter **18** Endocrine System

5. Why do you think that people continue behaviors, such as abuse of steroids and eating disorders, that have been demonstrated to harm them?

_____

_____

_____

6. When diabetes is discovered in an adolescent, the person often has difficulty adjusting to having the condition. Why do you think this might be true?

_____

_____

_____

Hormone Function

Hormones may be categorized according to the type of function they have in the body. These functions may stimulate other endocrine glands (tropic hormones), reproduction (sex hormones), or the building of tissues (anabolic hormones). Place the hormones into chart according to their function as described in Chapter 18 of the textbook.

ACTH
Aldosterone
Androgen
Antidiuretic hormone (ADH)
Calcitonin
Cortisol
Epinephrine
Estrogen
FSH
Glucagon
Insulin
Interstitial cell-stimulating hormone (ICSH)
Luteinizing hormone (LH)

Melatonin
Norepinephrine
Oxytocin
Parathyroid hormone
Parathyroid hormone
Progesterone
Prolactin
Somatotropic hormone (SH)
Testosterone
Thymosin
Thyroxine
Triiodothyronine
TSH

Topic (Target Other Endocrine Glands)	Sex (Target Reproductive Structures)	Anabolic (Stimulate Anabolism In Cells)

Endocrine Topics

Use the Internet to research one of the following topics. Write an essay, make a poster, or make a pamphlet that describes the topic.

Simeons Therapy (Human Chorionic Gonadotropin Diet)
Suggested Website

WebMD: http://www.webmd.com/diet/features/weight-loss-cure-dont-want-you-to-know

Steroid Abuse
Suggested Websites

SteroidAbuse.com: http://www.steroidabuse.com/steroid-abuse-in-sports.html
Department of Justice: http://www.deadiversion.usdoj.gov/pubs/brochures/steroids/professionals/index.html

Diabetes Mellitus
Suggested Websites

MedlinePlus: http://www.nlm.nih.gov/medlineplus/ency/article/001214.htm
Medscape: http://emedicine.medscape.com/article/919999-overview

Bovine Growth Hormone in Milk
Suggested Website

Wikipedia: http://en.wikipedia.org/wiki/Bovine_somatotropin

Endocrine Disruptors
Suggested Website

NIH: http://www.niehs.nih.gov/health/topics/agents/endocrine/index.cfm

Diabetes Risk Calculator

Use the following link to calculate your risk of developing diabetes. Write a paragraph to describe the things you can do to prevent it from occurring.

Suggested Website

American Diabetes Association: http://www.diabetes.org/diabetes-basics/prevention/diabetes-risk-test/

Essay

_____

_____

_____

_____

_____

_____

_____

_____

_____

_____

_____

_____

_____

_____

Essay (Cont'd)

19 Nervous System

VAPID VOCABULARY

Find the key terms in the word search puzzle and define them in the spaces provided.

```
C B E G O R L Y D D B T V I C E N Y
F E J T E I S C H E M I A M B B E N
R Y R F A P O C C J I P T P R J U J
A M L E E R A E M Z O D X U J H R O
X E E L B U E D W L P D Z L D S O E
X A I N A R M N Y B G T D S R S T P
A P B X I M O N E E L I N E S J R D
E J X U Y N E S W G B W P K D X A B
Y D Z U D U G R P J E R G C D O N A
I X V M R T I E S I P R P K X E S I
V E S I Y Q R U S K N Q Y L I K M T
I M T Z K N N Z I M T A L V I K I N
C I I W B Y H P A R G O L E Y M T E
S W F Y R H E P I X Y U T F Z Z T M
Y M L Y M C B R P V Y G L B L G E E
N I Q C L J A S O I S C H R D U R D
M F X R L Z D V Z T W T D W E C I M
S Y Z J W O F T N N Y Y Z U F H W D
```

1. Cerebrospinal fluid: _____

2. Dementia: _____

3. Epilepsy: _____

4. Impulse: _____

5. Intracranial: _____

6. Ischemia: _____

7. Meninges: _____

8. Myelography: _____

Continued

203

9. Neurotransmitter: _____

10. Polyneuritis: _____

11. Reflex: _____

12. Regenerate: _____

13. Senile: _____

ABBREVIATIONS

Match each of the following abbreviations with the phrase that best describes its meaning or function. Then write the phrase or name for each of the abbreviations in the spaces provided.

Abbreviation	Meaning or Function
1. _____ ANS	a. Brain and spinal cord
2. _____ CJD	b. Cranial and spinal nerves
3. _____ CNS	c. Damage to the spinal cord
4. _____ CVA	d. Examination of cerebrospinal fluid taken from the spinal cord
5. _____ CT	e. Little stroke
6. _____ LP	f. Mad cow disease
7. _____ MRI	g. Stroke
8. _____ PNS	h. Sympathetic and parasympathetic part of the peripheral nervous system
9. _____ SCI	i. Test using radio waves measure energy changes in cells
10. _____ TIA	j. X-ray that reconstructs sectional slices of the body

1. ANS: _____

2. CJD: _____

3. CNS: _____

4. CVA: _____

5. CT: _____

6. LP: _____

7. MRI: _____

8. PNS: _____

9. SCI: _____

10. TIA: _____

1. The function of the nervous system is to _ _ _ _ _, _ _ _ _ _ _ ◯ _ _ _, and
   _ _ _ _ _ _ _ to internal and external environmental changes to maintain a steady state in the body.

2. The central nervous system is made up of the _ _ ◯ _ _ and _ _ _ _ _ _ _ _ _ _ _.

3. The peripheral nervous system consists of 12 pairs of _ _ _ _ _ _ _ nerves and 31 pairs of
   _ _ _ _ _ _ nerves.

4. The _ _ _ _ _ _ _ _ ◯ _ nervous system has two parts, called the *sympathetic* system and the
   parasympathetic system.

5. The basic structural unit of the nervous system is the _ _ _ _ _, which consists of
   ◯ _ _ _ _ _ cells.

6. The neuron has three main parts, called the _ _ _ _ _ _ _ _ _ _, _ _ _ _, and
   _ _ _ _.

7. A ◯ _ _ _ _ _ _ is the space between two neurons.

8. The four major areas of the brain are the _ _ _ _ _ ◯ _ _, the diencephalon, the
   _ _ _ _ _ _ _ _ _ _ _, and the brain stem.

9. Two nervous system disorders that result from genetic causes are _ ◯ _ _
   _ _ _ _ _ _ _ _ and _ _ ◯ _ _ _ _ _ _ _ ' _ chorea.

10. The disorder of the nervous system called a *transient ischemic* _ _ _ _ _ ◯ may be an indicator of a
    more severe condition, called a _ _ _ _ _ _ _ _ _ ◯ _ _ _ _ _ accident.

Use the circled letters to form the answer to this jumble. Clue: What nervous system disorder has been treated with some success by implanting cells in the brain?

_ _ _ _ _ _ _ _ _ ' _

Identifying Structures and Functions of the Neuron

Use Figure 19-6 of the textbook to label the diagram of the neuron in Figure 19-1. In Table 19-1, describe the function of each part.

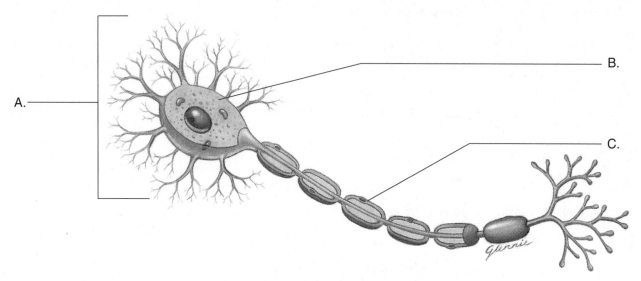

A.

B.

C.

Figure 19-1

TABLE 19-1   Structures and Functions of the Neuron

NEURON PART	MAIN FUNCTION
A.	
B.	
C.	

Identifying Structures and Functions of the Brain

Use Figure 19-8 of the textbook to color and label the diagram of the brain in Figure 19-2. In Table 19-2, describe the function of each part.

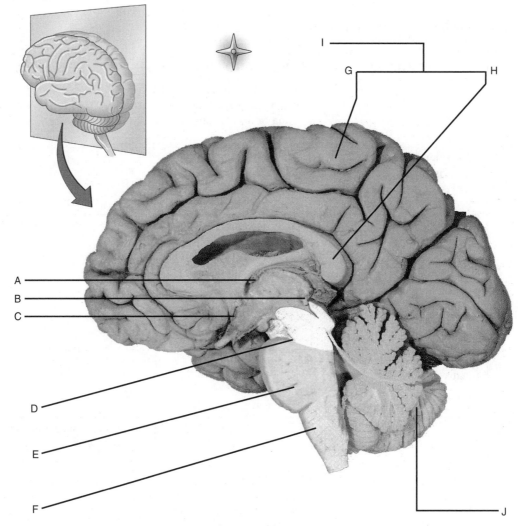

Figure 19-2

TABLE 19-2   Structures and Functions of the Brain

BRAIN PART	MAIN FUNCTION
Cerebellum	
Cerebrum	
Frontal lobe	
Medulla	
Midbrain	
Occipital lobe	
Parietal lobe	
Pons	
Spinal cord	
Temporal lobe	

Identifying Disorders of the Nervous System

Use the textbook to provide the missing information about nervous system disorders in Table 19-3. Note the name of the disorder, etiology (causing factor), signs and symptoms, and treatment and method of prevention (if any).

TABLE 19-3   Disorders of the Nervous System

DISORDER	ETIOLOGY	SIGNS AND SYMPTOMS	TREATMENT AND PREVENTION
		Degeneration of myelin sheath may cause double vision or loss of muscle control	
	Blood clot or vessel break causes ischemia in brain		
		Paralysis below the area of injury	
		Loss of memory and progressive impaired function	
	Bacteria, virus, or fungus		
			Medication, avoid triggers such as certain foods
		May range from sensory change to loss of responsiveness and tonic/clonic movement	

Applying Your Knowledge

1. One of the most common forms of mental retardation results from a genetic disorder that is caused by the presence of an extra chromosome. This condition is called _____.

2. When the brain is damaged by a lack of oxygen in one area, the condition may commonly be called

   _____.

3. Head pains due to stress are called _____ headaches, whereas those that result from vascular

   problems of unknown cause are called _____.

4. Swelling of membranes in the skull's cavities may lead to a third kind of headache, called a _____ headache.

5. One neurologic disorder that may be prevented by vaccination is _____.

Chapter **19** **Nervous System**

Assessing Neurologic Signs

One method used to quickly determine the level of function of the neurologic system is to assess the neurologic vital signs, or "neuro" signs. The following is the procedure for a short assessment of these functions. Read all of the directions before beginning this activity. Laboratory activities should be completed under the supervision of a qualified professional only.

Equipment and Supplies

Penlight

Directions

1. Work in pairs for this activity. One person acts as subject and the other as examiner throughout the activity. The roles may then be reversed.
2. Construct a chart to record the information needed to document the results of this activity. Place each type of assessment in the vertical column and "Right," "Left," and "Comments" as the horizontal column titles.
3. Observe the subject to determine the level of responsiveness. Level of responsiveness may be described in one of the following terms:
   - *Alert:* Aware of surroundings and environmental stimuli; responds to verbal stimulus, such as talking.
   - *Lethargic:* May be made aware of environmental stimuli with assistance; responds to loud verbal stimuli or touch.
   - *Stuporous:* Does not respond to environmental stimuli; may be roused with return to sleepwalk state quickly; responds to touch and pain stimuli.
   - *Comatose:* Does not respond to any stimuli.
4. Record the level of responsiveness of the subject:

_____

5. Determine the orientation of the subject by asking questions that assess awareness of person, place, and time. The questions should require more than a "yes" or "no" answer to determine whether the answer is appropriate. For example:
   - "Tell me your name, please" asks for orientation of person. It would be acceptable for the person to name a relative if asked for that information.
   - "What day of the week is it?" asks for orientation to time. This question may be difficult for someone who has been hospitalized for awhile. Knowing the year or the name of the current president would be acceptable in this and some other circumstances.
   - "Tell me the name of this facility" asks for orientation to place. Knowing the city or similar information would be acceptable in these and some other situations.
       Normal orientation is "oriented × 3," or to all three areas of inquiry. If the person is not oriented in one or more of the areas, an example of the incorrect response should be recorded. If the subject cannot answer or gives incorrect responses, the correct information should be given to the subject to prevent anxiety.
6. Record the orientation of the subject:

_____

7. Assess the response of the pupils to light. Observe the pupils of both eyes. They should be equal in size. Turn on a small flashlight or penlight. Bring the light from the side of the face to shine into the center of the subject's right eye, keeping the flashlight about 6 inches away from the face. Observe the pupils of both eyes as the light nears the right eye. The pupils of both eyes should contract quickly and equally. Remove the light. The pupils should return to their original size quickly and equally. Repeat the exercise by shining the light in the left eye. This result is recorded as PEERL or PERRLA (pupils equal in size and equally reactive to light).
8. Record the pupil responses:

_____

9. Assess the function of facial nerves and muscles. Instruct the subject to stick out the tongue as far as possible. The tongue should extend in a symmetrical manner on both sides.
10. Record the facial muscle response:

_____

11. Assess the strength and equality of nerve and muscle response of the hands. Instruct the subject to grip and squeeze the index and middle finger of both of your hands as hard as possible until asked to stop. The grips of the subject should be equal and strong.

12. Record the grip responses:

_____

13. Assess the strength and equality of the nerve and muscle response of the feet. For this assessment, the subject should be lying down or sitting with the legs extended. Place one arm across the soles of the subject's feet, and instruct the subject to push as hard as possible with both feet. The push response of the subject's feet should be equal and strong.

14. Record the push responses:

_____

Drawing Conclusions

1. When neurologic vital signs are taken every 15 minutes, it is necessary to vary the questions slightly. It is also important to explain to the client that the procedure will be repeated. What might the client think if the procedure were repeated several times without explanation?

_____

_____

_____

2. Clients are given more than one chance to answer questions of orientation correctly. This is especially important if the client is awakened for the assessment. Why would this be important?

_____

_____

_____

3. A person may have a level of responsiveness of being alert and an orientation of being confused. How would this appear in the neurologic assessment?

_____

_____

_____

4. Which cranial nerve is being assessed when the pupil response is tested?

_____

5. Why is it necessary to test the pupil response by shining the light into each eye separately?

_____

_____

_____

6. List three factors that might influence the results of the pupil response assessment.

_____

_____

_____

Assessing Cranial Nerve Functions

One of the methods used to assess neurologic function tests the function of the cranial nerves. Use the textbook to list each of the 12 cranial nerves and their functions in Table 19-4. Then complete the laboratory activity. Read all of the directions before beginning this activity. Laboratory activities should be completed under the supervision of a qualified professional only.

TABLE 19-4   Cranial Nerve Functions

CRANIAL NERVE	MAIN FUNCTION
I.	
II.	
III.	
IV.	
V.	
VI.	
VII.	
VIII.	
IX.	
X.	
XI.	
XII.	

Equipment and Supplies

Alarm clock
Audiogram (optional)
Containers of items for identification of odor
Cotton swabs
Items for assessment of taste
Penlight
Snellen chart
Tongue depressor

Directions

1. Work in pairs for this activity. One person acts as the subject and the other as the examiner throughout the activity. The roles may then be reversed.
2. Construct a chart on which to record the results of this activity.
3. To assess the function of the first cranial nerve, have the subject close both eyes and block one nostril. Present items for identification that have a familiar odor. Items to be smelled should be kept in sealed containers before and after use. Some examples of items for identification include coffee, soap, peanut butter, and vanilla. Repeat the process for the other nostril. Record the results of the assessment in your chart.
4. The second cranial nerve can be tested using an eye chart to determine visual acuity. The procedure for determining visual acuity is presented in Chapter 25 of the textbook. Record the visual acuity of each eye separately and of the two eyes together in your chart.
5. The third, fourth, and sixth cranial nerves can be tested at the same time, because they all regulate eye movement. The subject may demonstrate this function by following the movement of your finger in lateral and vertical directions. Eye movement should be the same with both eyes. Record the results of the assessment in your chart.
6. The motor function of the fifth cranial nerve can be assessed with the subject biting down on the teeth as hard as possible. The muscles of the jaw should be observed to be tight and equal in size. The sensory function of this nerve can be assessed for the equal sensation of temperature and touch on both sides of the face. Record the results of the assessment in your chart.

7. The seventh cranial nerve has both sensory and motor function. The motor function controls facial expression. To assess this nerve, have the subject frown, smile widely, and puff out the cheeks. The muscle movements should appear equal in strength and symmetry. Record the results of the assessment in your chart.

8. The eighth cranial nerve can be assessed using the audiogram to perform a hearing test. The function may also be assessed in a rough manner by using a small, winding alarm clock. The subject should be able to hear the ticking of the clock from 20 feet away. Test each ear separately by blocking one at a time and then test the two ears together. Record the results of the assessment in your chart.

9. The ninth and tenth cranial nerves may be assessed at the same time. Part of the function of the ninth cranial nerve is taste on the posterior tongue. It may be tested in the manner described in Chapter 20 of the workbook. However, swallowing and the gag reflex demonstrate the motor function of these nerves. When an object touches the posterior pharynx, the palate should elevate and retract upward. A clean tongue depressor may be used with care to prevent injury to the soft tissues of the mouth in this assessment. Record the results of the assessment in your chart.

10. The eleventh cranial nerve activates the movement of the trapezius and sternocleidomastoid muscles. To assess this function, have the subject turn the head to one side and push the chin in the same direction against the resistance of your hand. The sternocleidomastoid muscle in the neck should stand out visibly with this effort. The trapezius muscle can be assessed in the same manner. Place your hand on the subject's shoulders and have the person shrug or lift the shoulders against your hands. The force of the resistance against your hands should be strong. Record the results of the assessment in your chart.

11. The twelfth cranial nerve may be assessed by observing the movement of the tongue. Have the subject stick out the tongue. It should extend in a symmetrical manner. Record the results of the assessment in your chart.

Drawing Conclusions

1. Why must the assessments be performed separately for both sides of the body?

_____

_____

_____

2. In the assessment of the olfactory nerve, why is it important to keep the containers sealed tightly before and after being used for assessment?

_____

_____

_____

3. Why is it necessary to test both the motor and sensory function of the trigeminal, facial, glossopharyngeal, and vagal cranial nerves?

_____

_____

_____

4. Are the results of the assessment within the normal range?

_____

_____

_____

5. List three factors that might influence the results of this activity.

_____

_____

_____

Brain Dominance

Most people are either right- or left-handed. That is because one side of the brain dominates its use. Perform the following activities to complete Table 19-5 by placing a check in the right or left column.

TABLE 19-5   Brain Dominance

PART OF BODY	TEST	RIGHT	LEFT
Hand	Write name		
Hand	Use scissors		
Hand	Throw ball		
Hand	Drink from cup		
Hand	Eat using fork		
Foot	Kick ball		
Foot	Step up stair		
Foot	Step on object		
Eye	Look in tube		
Eye	Sight a finger		
Eye	Look through hole		
Ear	Listen to whisper		
Ear	Listen to box		
Ear	Listen through wall		

Equipment

Pen, pencil, paper
Scissors
Ball
Cup of water
Stairs
Coin
Small tube
Paper with small hole
Small box with mystery item inside

Directions

1. Work in pairs to perform this activity.
2. Observe your partner while he or she performs each of the following activities. Using Table 19-5, record which hand is used.
   - Writing his or her name
   - Cutting with scissors
   - Throwing a ball
   - Eating with a fork
   - Drinking from a cup
3. Observe your partner while he or she performs each of the following activities. Using Table 19-5, record which foot is used.
   - Kicking a ball
   - Stepping up on stairs
   - Stepping on a coin

4. Observe your partner while he or she performs each of the following activities. Using Table 19-5, record which eye is used.
   - Looking through a tube
   - "Sighting" an object (This is determined by holding a finger up in alignment with a distant object, such as a clock, with both eyes open. When one eye is closed, the object will "jump" or appear to move. Record which eye is used when the object does not appear to move.)
   - Looking through a small hole in a piece of paper
5. Observe your partner while he or she performs each of the following activities. Using Table 19-5, record which ear is used.
   - Listens to a whisper
   - Tries to identify an unknown object in a box by sound
   - Tries to listen through a wall

Drawing Conclusions

1. Which side of your brain is more dominant?

_____

2. Explain why someone might use the right hand to throw a ball and use the left hand to eat with a fork.

_____

_____

_____

3. What activities, when considered alone, might not indicate the brain dominance?

_____

_____

_____

CRITICAL THINKING

Coma Therapy

Sensory stimulation is used with great success to treat people in comas. Some examples of stimulation include playing loud music and applying hot peppers and vinegar to the tongue. Ammonia is used to activate the sense of smell. Conversation is held in the room and directed to the comatose individual to stimulate the brain's responses. This type of aggressive coma therapy is based on the theory that continual stimulation of the senses helps the brain remember these stimulants and how to respond to them. With aggressive therapy, coma clients receive 8 hours of intensive activity each day, including physical, occupational, and speech therapy.

Examining the Evidence

1. The cost of intensive coma therapy is high. How do you think this cost might compare with the cost of maintaining someone in a coma for a long period of time?

_____

_____

_____

2. The theory behind aggressive stimulation of the senses for a comatose client assumes that the brain is able to assess and respond to stimuli even if no reaction is seen. Describe at least one other situation or state in which a person is normally unresponsive to stimuli.

_____

_____

_____

214

3. If the theory about the brain's responses is proven to be true, how might that alter the care of the client in the state you described in question 2?

_____

_____

_____

Recognizing Reflexes

Fill in Table 19-6 by indicating the reflex that occurs as a result of the indicated stimulus.

TABLE 19-6   Reflexes

STIMULUS	RESULTING REFLEX ACTION
1. Feeling cold and wet	
2. Feeling hot	
3. Coming up to the surface after swimming underwater	
4. Swallowing something into the trachea	
5. Loud, unexpected noise	
6. Getting a foreign particle in the eye	
7. Inhaling pepper	
8. Bright light	
9. Being tickled	
10. Stepping on a tack	

INTERNET ACTIVITIES

Nervous System Topics

Use the Internet to research one of the following topics. Write an essay, make a poster, or make a pamphlet that describes the topic.

College Dorm Meningitis
Suggested Websites

CDC: http://www.cdc.gov/mmwr/preview/mmwrhtml/rr4907a2.htm
KidsHealth: http://kidshealth.org/parent/infections/lung/meningitis.html

Spinal Cord Injury Research
Suggested Website

Reeve Foundation: http://www.christopherreeve.org/site/c.ddJFKRNoFiG/b.4343879/k.D323/Research.htm

Stroke Treatment
Suggested Website

WebMD: http://www.webmd.com/stroke/guide/stroke-treatment-overview

Brain Activities

Complete the online activities to determine your neurologic type and ability.
   BBC Science & Nature Memory Survey: http://www.bbc.co.uk/science/humanbody/mind/surveys/memory/
   BBC Science & Nature Perception Survey:
   http://www.bbc.co.uk/science/humanbody/mind/surveys/synaesthesia/see/

Essay

20 Sensory System

VAPID VOCABULARY

Find the key terms in the word search puzzle and define them in the spaces provided.

```
L  F  D  F  L  N  V  N  A  N  I  Y  N  K  Q
R  C  F  M  K  I  F  E  C  O  Y  R  H  W  C
R  A  I  Q  S  O  G  G  C  I  G  O  V  S  P
Y  L  L  I  O  R  J  A  O  T  U  T  N  T  M
E  R  O  U  E  T  U  L  M  C  S  I  H  I  U
W  N  O  V  C  X  H  A  M  A  T  D  R  M  G
X  E  N  T  M  O  E  K  O  R  A  U  G  U  A
T  O  M  V  C  Y  A  G  D  F  T  A  L  L  Z
C  P  Z  I  H  A  Y  R  A  E  O  L  A  U  R
V  G  R  U  I  E  F  U  T  R  R  H  M  S  C
Z  Z  Z  C  A  Y  C  L  I  N  Y  F  Q  R  M
R  E  C  E  P  T  O  R  O  O  I  B  A  Y  X
C  A  P  X  C  U  T  A  N  E  O  U  S  M  G
M  U  I  R  B  I  L  I  U  Q  E  H  C  F  A
E  C  H  T  N  I  R  Y  B  A  L  N  I  R  S
```

1. Accommodation: _____

2. Auditory: _____

3. Converge: _____

4. Cutaneous: _____

5. Equilibrium: _____

6. Gustatory: _____

7. Intraocular: _____

8. Labyrinth: _____

9. Olfactory: _____

10. Receptor: _____

Continued

11. Refraction: _____

12. Stimulus: _____

13. Vision: _____

ABBREVIATIONS

Match each of the following abbreviations with the phrase that best describes its meaning or function. Then write the phrase or name for each of the abbreviations in the spaces provided.

Abbreviation	**Meaning or Function**
1. _____ 20/10	a. Better than normal vision
2. _____ 20/20	b. Common treatment is scleral buckle to restore vision
3. _____ 20/30	c. Ear infection
4. _____ CI	d. Normal vision
5. _____ dB	e. Surgical procedure for myopia correction
6. _____ Hg	f. Surgical procedure for restoring hearing
7. _____ LASIK	g. Surgical procedure that uses lasers to improve vision
8. _____ OM	h. Unit of measurement for pressure in the eye
9. _____ RD	i. Unit of measurement for loudness
10. _____ RK	j. Worse than normal vision

1. 20/10: _____

2. 20/20: _____

3. 20/30: _____

4. CI: _____

5. dB: _____

6. Hg: _____

7. LASIK: _____

8. OM: _____

9. RD: _____

10. RK: _____

1. The sensory system consists of receptors in specialized cells and organs that perceive changes in the

   _ _ _ _ _ _ _ _ _ and _ _ Ⓞ _ _ _ _ _ environment.

2. Specialized cells in the retina, called _ _ _ Ⓞ and Ⓞ _ _ _ _, absorb the light.

3. The _ _ _ Ⓞ _ _ _ _ sense is the primary function of the ear; a second function is to help

   maintain _ _ _ _ _ _ _ _ _ _ _ _.

4. Specialized cells located in _ _ _ Ⓞ _ _ _ _ _ _ _ on the tongue or

   Ⓞ _ _ _ _ _ _ _ _ _ _ _ _ _ perceive taste.

5. The olfactory sense originates in cells in the nose, which immediately transmit impulses to the brain through the

   olfactory _ _ _ Ⓞ _ _ _ _ _ _ Ⓞ _ _.

6. The _ Ⓞ _ _ _ _ _ _ _ senses of the skin perceive touch, pressure, temperature, and pain

   through _ Ⓞ _ _ specialized cells located in the skin.

7. A disorder of the sensory system that is often related to diabetes mellitus is _ _ _ _ _ _ _ _

   _ _ _ _ _ _ _ _ _ _ _.

8. Two conditions of the eye that are often corrected with glasses are _ _ _ _ _ _ _ Ⓞ _ and

   _ _ _ _ _ _.

9. A common disorder of vision that occurs with aging is _ _ _ _ _ _ Ⓞ _ _ _.

10. Most people do not notice a loss in hearing until they cannot understand _ _ _ _ _ _

    _ _ Ⓞ _ _ _ _ _ Ⓞ _ _ _.

   Use the circled letters to form the answer to this jumble. Clue: What is a common bacterial or viral eye infection that causes reddening of the eyelids and is extremely contagious?

   _ _ _ _ _ _ _ _ _ _ _ _ _ _ _

Identifying Structures and Functions of the Eye

Use Figure 20-1 of the textbook to label the diagram of the eye in Figure 20-1. In the spaces provided in Table 20-1, describe the function of each part.

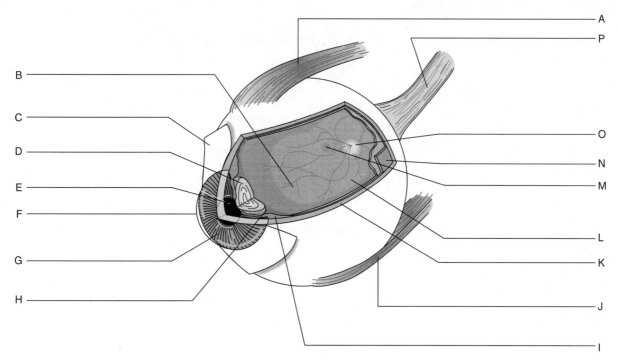

Figure 20-1

TABLE 20-1   Structures and Functions of the Eye

EYE PART	MAIN FUNCTION
Anterior cavity	
Choroid coat	
Ciliary muscle	
Conjunctiva	
Cornea	
Iris	
Lens	
Optic nerve	
Posterior cavity	
Pupil	
Retina	
Sclera	
Suspensory ligaments	

Identifying Structures and Functions of the Ear

Use Figure 20-3 of the textbook to color and label the diagram of the ear in Figure 20-2. Use different colors to indicate structures of the external, middle, and inner ear. In the spaces provided in Table 20-2, describe the function of each part.

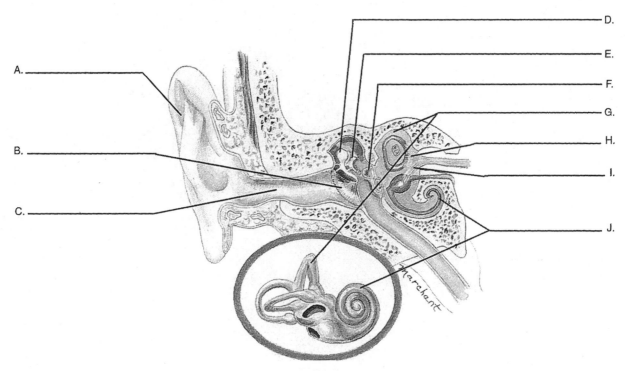

Figure 20-2

TABLE 20-2   Structures and Functions of the Ear

EAR PART	MAIN FUNCTION
Auditory canal	
Cochlea	
Incus	
Malleus	
Oval window	
Pinna	
Semicircular canal	
Stapes	
Tympanic membrane	
Vestibule	

Identifying Structures and Functions of the Nose

Use Figure 20-5 of the textbook to label the diagram of the nose in Figure 20-3. In the spaces provided in Table 20-3, describe the function of each part.

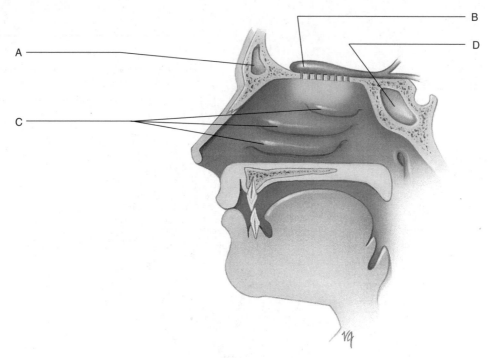

Figure 20-3

TABLE 20-3   Structures and Functions of the Nose

NOSE PART	MAIN FUNCTION
Frontal sinus	
Nasal turbinate	
Olfactory bulb	
Sphenoid sinus	

Identifying Structures and Functions of the Skin

Use Figure 20-6 in the textbook to label the diagram of the skin in Figure 20-4. In the spaces provided in Table 20-4, describe the function of each part.

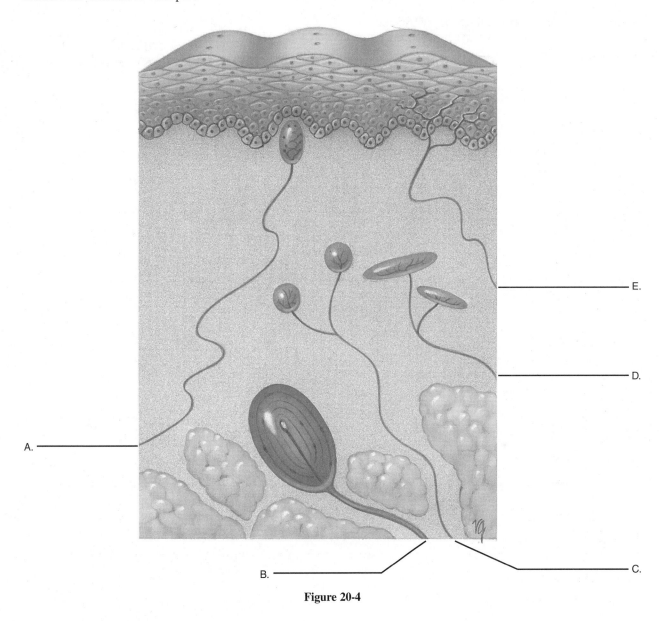

Figure 20-4

TABLE 20-4   Structures and Functions of the Skin

SKIN PART	MAIN FUNCTION
End-bulb of Krause	
Meissner's corpuscles	
Pacinian corpuscles	
Pain receptor	
Ruffini's corpuscles	

Chapter **20** **Sensory System**

Identifying Disorders of the Sensory System

Use the textbook to provide the missing information about sensory system disorders in Table 20-5. Note the name of the disorder, etiology (causing factor), signs and symptoms, and treatment and method of prevention (if any).

TABLE 20-5   Disorders of the Sensory System

DISORDER	ETIOLOGY	SIGNS AND SYMPTOMS	TREATMENT AND PREVENTION
			Antibiotics, may include myringotomy
	Genetic, defect on X chromosome		
		Increased intraocular pressure, may cause pain or no symptoms	
	Congenital defect of eyeball		
	Inflammation of the cavity of the cranium, nasal obstruction		
		Clouding of the lens of the eye leading to blurred or partial vision	
		Inflammation and reddening of eyelids and sclera with pus formation, extremely contagious	

Applying Your Knowledge

1. Hearing loss may result from a problem in _____ or _____.

2. The correct term for a nosebleed is _____. One cause may be _____.

3. Children with the infection called _____ may be treated by the insertion of tubes to drain the middle ear.

4. One symptom that may be caused by sinus, chemical, viral, or allergic irritation may be _____.

5. A stye is caused by a bacterial infection in the _____ of the eyelid.

INVESTIGATIONS

Demonstrating Taste Ability

Read all of the directions before beginning this activity. Although receptors for taste are located on all surfaces of the tongue, the understanding of taste also depends on the smell and texture of food. Laboratory activities should be completed under the supervision of a qualified professional only.

224

Equipment and Supplies

Blindfold
Three small pieces of peeled apple in a paper bag
Three small pieces of peeled potato in the same paper bag
Nose plug

Directions

1. Work in pairs for this activity. One person acts as the subject and the other as the examiner throughout the activity. The roles may then be reversed.
2. Place the nose plug and blindfold on one person.
3. Randomly choose a small piece of apple or potato from the paper bag and try to identify it by taste alone.
4. Repeat until all items from the paper bag have been identified.
5. Reverse roles and repeat the activity.

Drawing Conclusions

1. How many of the pieces of food did you and your partner identify correctly?

_____

_____

_____

2. In what other circumstance would the taste of food be difficult to interpret?

_____

_____

_____

3. What other foods might confuse someone with limited ability to smell?

_____

_____

_____

Demonstrating Skin Sensitivity

Read all of the directions before beginning this activity. Although receptors for touch are located on all surfaces of the body, the type and frequency of these receptors vary. Laboratory activities should be completed under the supervision of a qualified professional only.

Equipment and Supplies

Blindfold
Bristles of varied size

Directions

1. Work in pairs for this activity. One person acts as the subject and the other as the examiner throughout the activity. The roles may then be reversed.
2. The smallest stimulus that produces a response of a neuron is called the *threshold stimulus*. To determine the threshold stimulus, blindfold the subject. Then gently touch the subject's fingertip with a small bristle until it bends. The subject should indicate whether the bristle can be felt.
3. Repeat step 1 using three different bristles of varied thicknesses. Try each bristle randomly, using each type at least five times. Record the results of the activity in Table 20-6.
4. Repeat the procedure, touching the bristles to the back of the subject's hand. Record the results of this activity in Table 20-7.
5. Repeat the procedure, touching the bristles to the subject's forearm. Record the results of this activity in Table 20-8.
6. Repeat the procedure, touching the back of the subject's neck with the bristles. Record the results of this activity in Table 20-9.
7. Exchange roles and repeat the activity.

225

TABLE 20-6 Fingertip

BRISTLE	SM	MED	LG
Trial 1			
Trial 2			
Trial 3			
Trial 4			
Trial 5			

TABLE 20-7 Back of the Hand

BRISTLE	SM	MED	LG
Trial 1			
Trial 2			
Trial 3			
Trial 4			
Trial 5			

TABLE 20-8 Forearm

BRISTLE	SM	MED	LG
Trial 1			
Trial 2			
Trial 3			
Trial 4			
Trial 5			

TABLE 20-9 Back of the Neck

BRISTLE	SM	MED	LG
Trial 1			
Trial 2			
Trial 3			
Trial 4			
Trial 5			

Drawing Conclusions

1. Which part of the body tested has the lowest threshold of sensitivity (which felt the thinnest bristle most frequently)?

_____

2. Which part of the body tested has the highest threshold of sensitivity (which felt the thinnest bristles least frequently)?

_____

3. Based on your observations, hypothesize why some areas of the skin are more sensitive than others.

_____

_____

_____

CRITICAL THINKING

Patterns of Sleep

About one-third of a human life is spent sleeping. Sleeping is defined as the recurrent, normal condition of unresponsiveness with limited movement. Scientists do not agree on the reason that sleep occurs, but all agree that it is necessary for a healthy life. The theories that have been suggested to explain the need for sleep include:
- To remove the buildup of metabolic waste from the brain
- To allow rest of the nerve tissues
- To remove excess hormones from the body

Research into sleep patterns and disorders is a relatively new field. The time spent sleeping has been divided into five stages based on the brain's wave patterns. Drowsiness or relaxed wakefulness precedes but is not considered part of sleep. During this time the brain produces alpha waves, and images may occur in the brain. These images are not considered dreams. The stages of sleep are found in Table 20-10.

TABLE 20-10

STAGE	DESCRIPTION	BRAIN WAVE PATTERN	LENGTH	% OF SLEEP
Stage 1	Lightest sleep	Reduced alpha waves	1–2 min	
Stage 2	Light sleep	Frequent, regular waves	5–10 min	50%
Stage 3		Transition to delta waves	10 min	
Stage 4	Deep sleep	Delta waves	5–15 min	
Stage 5	REM or dream sleep		45 min	20%–25%

Normally, a person passes through the stages of sleep several times during a sleep cycle. At the end of each cycle, the brain wave activity resembles light sleep and rapid eye movement (REM) can be observed. This part of sleep is called *dream sleep*. The first period of REM sleep is the shortest, with each period becoming longer. The REM stage may last as long as 45 minutes before waking occurs. Regardless of whether the dreams are remembered, every person has three to five REM periods each night.

The amount of sleep necessary varies among individuals. Generally, newborns and infants need 14 to 20 hours of sleep. Young children need 12 to 14 hours of sleep. Adults usually need 7 to 9 hours in each 24-hour period. Sleep deprivation leads to a decrease in performance, irritability, agitation, tremors, lack of attention, and lethargy. Over a long period, lack of sleep can lead to brain damage and death. Sleep disorders are called parasomnias. The following is a description of several types of sleep patterns.

Insomnia is the inability to sleep. It is usually a symptom of another disorder. Insomniacs fall into three categories: some have difficulty falling asleep, others have trouble staying asleep, and still others awaken early. Generally, insomnia is caused by overstimulation due to anxiety, stress, or stimulants.

Hypersomnia is the condition in which a person sleeps 16 to 18 hours a day. This condition may be acute or chronic in nature. It often occurs with uremia, increased intracranial pressure, diabetic acidosis, or hypothyroidism. It may also occur as a reaction to stress.

Sleep apnea is a disorder that most often occurs in middle-aged men who are overweight and have high blood pressure. The person experiencing sleep apnea generally snores and then stops breathing for 30 to 40 seconds. The epiglottis is believed to fall back into the throat, closing the airway. The condition can be life threatening.

Enuresis, or bed wetting, has no clear-cut cause. Restricting fluid intake several hours before sleeping helps control the condition.

Somnambulism is commonly known as sleepwalking. It is seen most often in children, who eventually outgrow it. People who are sleepwalking are easily awakened and are not dreaming during this stage of sleep.

Talking in one's sleep is very common; almost everyone talks while asleep at some time.

Bruxism is grinding of the teeth that occurs during sleep. This condition may cause discomfort and damage to the teeth. Appliances or mouth guards may be worn to protect the teeth.

Night terrors and nightmares may become serious sleep disorders. The autonomic nervous system actually produces stress responses in the body during night terrors.

Narcolepsy is a form of epilepsy in which sleep occurs regardless of the person's position or activity. It is commonly called a sleep attack. Narcolepsy may often be controlled with medication.

Sleep may be induced with drugs that include sedatives. Sedatives, alcohol, tranquilizers, hypnotics, and amphetamines are drugs that alter the sleep pattern. When one of these drugs has been taken on a regular basis, rebound nightmares occur when the drug is stopped. It takes 3 to 5 weeks for the sleep cycle to return to normal once it has been altered.

Examining the Evidence

1. How much sleep is needed by an adolescent person?

_____

2. List five signs and symptoms that may indicate an inadequate amount of sleep.

_____

_____

_____

3. Why is sleep apnea life threatening?

_____

_____

_____

Issues of Hearing Loss

Normally, the human ear can distinguish or separate more than 350,000 different sounds. It is the most complex and efficient sensory organ. In the United States, hearing loss is the fourth most prevalent chronic physical disability. About one in eight Americans have some hearing loss during a lifetime.

Examining the Evidence

1. List three ways in which an adolescent's life would be altered if a serious hearing loss occurred.

_____

_____

_____

2. List three methods that might be used to help someone with a serious hearing loss understand procedures during a health examination or treatment.

_____

_____

_____

3. List three methods that might be used to preserve hearing later in life.

_____

_____

_____

INTERNET ACTIVITIES

Sensory System Topics

Use the Internet to research one of the following topics related to the sensory system. Write an essay, make a poster, or make a pamphlet that describes the topic.

Deaf Culture and Communities

Suggested Websites

Deaf Culture Online: http://www.deaf-culture-online.com/deafculture.html
ASL Info.com: http://www.aslinfo.com/deafculture.cfm

Noise Pollution

Suggested Websites

Quiet Org: http://www.quiet.org/faq.htm
Noise Pollution Clearinghouse: http://www.nonoise.org/
Kids Health: http://kidshealth.org/teen/diseases_conditions/sight/hearing_impairment.html
EPA: http://www.epa.gov/air/noise.html

Interactive Sensory System Activities

Use the Internet to explore some activities that demonstrate and test the function of the sensory system.

Suggested Websites

Neuroscience for Kids—Brain Games: http://faculty.washington.edu/chudler/chgames.html
Eye Digest: http://www.agingeye.net/visionbasics/healthyvision.php

Essay

_____

_____

_____

_____

_____

_____

_____

_____

_____

_____

_____

_____

_____

_____

_____

_____

229

Essay (Cont'd)

21 Reproductive System

VAPID VOCABULARY

Find the key terms in the word search puzzle and define them in the spaces provided.

```
I  H  F  G  Z  X  V  I  M  P  S  E  R  E  D
R  O  A  A  U  H  V  Q  B  I  H  C  L  N  W
M  H  E  Z  H  V  P  V  P  K  I  C  K  W  X
J  A  A  F  F  N  R  Z  G  S  Y  Z  M  D  Z
N  H  M  N  I  N  T  E  R  C  O  U  R  S  E
J  O  J  M  F  B  S  Z  L  P  C  C  G  E  L
M  G  I  W  O  T  R  A  L  I  Y  O  E  H  I
R  O  F  T  A  G  U  O  P  Y  S  N  N  T  T
M  G  S  T  A  R  R  O  I  T  W  C  I  Y  C
O  T  I  Z  T  L  T  A  E  D  E  E  T  K  E
Z  O  P  S  Q  C  U  R  P  D  O  P  A  O  R
N  C  N  I  E  Q  I  V  Q  H  Z  T  L  L  E
F  E  R  T  I  L  E  I  O  A  Y  I  Z  G  S
M  M  V  S  E  S  N  E  M  J  Q  O  B  J  A
N  O  I  T  A  T  C  A  L  B  A  N  A  X  G
```

1. Conception: _____

2. Ectopic: _____

3. Erectile: _____

4. Fertile: _____

5. Fibroid: _____

6. Genital: _____

7. Gestation: _____

8. Intercourse: _____

9. Lactation: _____

10. Mammography: _____

11. Menses: _____

Continued

231

12. Menstrual cycle: _____

13. Ovulation: _____

14. Sterile: _____

ABBREVIATIONS

Match each of the following abbreviations with the phrase that best describes its meaning or function. Then write the phrase or name for each of the abbreviations in the spaces provided.

Abbreviation	**Meaning or Function**
1. _____ ART	a. Collection of 150 symptoms related to the menstrual cycle
2. _____ FAS	b. Common, chronic condition that results from infection of reproductive organs
3. _____ GIFT	c. Diseases that are transmitted by sexual activity
4. _____ HSV-2	d. Genital warts
5. _____ HPV	e. Group of physical and mental birth defects resulting from alcohol crossing the placenta
6. _____ IVF	f. Severe form of PMS
7. _____ PID	g. Techniques used to increase reproduction
8. _____ PMDD	h. Test tube fertilization
9. _____ PMS	i. Type of ART involving injection of fertilized sperm into the fallopian tube
10. _____ STI	j. Virus that may lead to cervical cancer and for which there is a vaccine

1. ART: _____

2. FAS: _____

3. GIFT: _____

4. HSV-2: _____

5. HPV: _____

6. IVF: _____

7. PID: _____

8. PMDD: _____

9. PMS: _____

10. STI: _____

1. The function of the reproductive system is to produce _ _ _ _ _ ◯ _ _ _.

2. The reproductive organs of both the male and female produce sex cells called _ _ ◯ _ _ _ _.

3. The _ _ _ _ _ ◯ _ _ _   _ _ _ _ _ transport the mature ovum from the ovary to the uterus.

4. The _ _ _ _ _ ◯ is implanted in the uterus after conception.

5. Growth of an offspring in the uterus lasts about _ _ _   _ _ _ ◯ (9 months), or through the period of pregnancy.

6. A baby born before the thirty-seventh week of pregnancy is considered to be ◯ _ _ _ _ _ _ _ _ _.

7. Many abnormalities of the breasts and testes may be discovered by
◯ _ _ _ -_ ◯ _ _ _ _ _ _   _ _ _.

8. Tests that can be used to detect abnormalities of the fetus during gestation include
_ _ _ _ _ _ _ ◯ _ _ _ _ _ _, ultrasonography,
and _ ◯ _ _ _ _ _ _ _ villus sampling.

9. Three sexually transmitted diseases that are caused by bacteria are _ _ ◯ _ _ _ _ ◯ _, syphilis,
and _ _ _ _ _ _ _ _ _.

10. A common cause of _ _ _ ◯ _ _ _ _ _ _ _ is damage to the fallopian tubes as a result of pelvic inflammatory disease.

Use the circled letters to form the answer to this jumble. Clue: What is a common disorder of the reproductive system that results from a viral infection and has no cure?

_ _ _ _ _ _   _ _ _ _ _ _

Identifying Structures and Functions of the Male Reproductive System

Use Figure 21-2 in the textbook to color and label the diagram of the male reproductive system in Figure 21-1. In the spaces provided in Table 21-1, describe the function of each part.

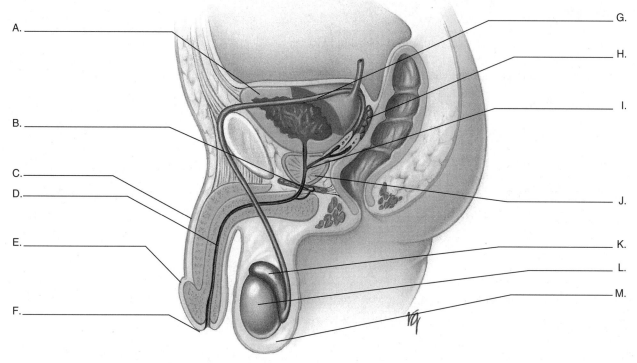

A.

B.

C.

D.

E.

F.

G.

H.

I.

J.

K.

L.

M.

Figure 21-1

TABLE 21-1 Structures and Functions of the Male Reproductive System

REPRODUCTIVE PART	MAIN FUNCTION
Cowper's gland	
Ejaculatory duct	
Epididymis	
Glans penis	
Penis	
Prostate gland	
Scrotum	
Seminal vesicle	
Testis	
Urethra	
Urinary bladder	
Urinary meatus	
Vas deferens	

Identifying Structures and Functions of the Female Reproductive System

Use Figure 21-4 of the textbook to color and label the diagrams of the female reproductive system in Figure 21-2. In the spaces provided in Table 21-2, describe the function of each part.

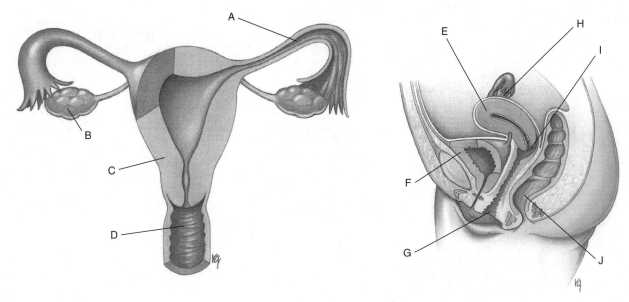

Figure 21-2

A _____   F _____

B _____   G _____

C _____   H _____

D _____   I _____

E _____   J _____

TABLE 21-2 Structures and Functions of the Female Reproductive System

REPRODUCTIVE PART	MAIN FUNCTION
Cervix	
Fallopian tube	
Ovary	
Rectum	
Urinary bladder	
Uterus	
Vagina	

Identifying Disorders of the Reproductive System

Use the textbook to provide the missing information about reproductive system disorders in Table 21-3. Note the name of the disorder, etiology (causing factor), signs and symptoms, and treatment and method of prevention (if any).

TABLE 21-3   Disorders of the Reproductive System

DISORDER	ETIOLOGY	SIGNS AND SYMPTOMS	TREATMENT AND PREVENTION
	Chronic infection such as gonorrhea or chlamydia		
		Blisters that develop into open painful sores appearing in episodes	
		Painless sores, fever, swollen glands, rash, nervous system damage	
	Alcohol consumption by mother of unborn baby		
		Painful urination, white to yellowish green discharge from urethra, may have no symptoms in women	
			Surgical removal, freezing, chemical, or electrical burning
	Hormonal or biochemical imbalance, poor nutrition		

Applying Your Knowledge

1. The most common sexually transmitted disease, called _____, is one of several that may have no symptoms in women. Another that may have no symptoms in women is called _____.

2. The child that will be affected by erythroblastosis fetalis is the _____ or later.

3. The ratio of people who develop genital warts after contact with them is _____.

4. When a mother drinks alcohol during pregnancy, the effects on the fetus may be mental or physical. The condition called _____ _____ can be cured by _____.

5. It is estimated that more than 100,000 women become infertile each year by the condition called

   _____ _____ _____. This condition is

   developed by _____ women annually.

INVESTIGATIONS

See the Evolve website for an optional activity on demonstrating embryo development.

CRITICAL THINKING

Ethical Issues of Reproduction

Newspaper headlines demonstrate the complexity of the ethical issues surrounding innovations in reproduction. How a person feels about these issues is a result of past experience, religious beliefs, education, and many other factors. The following questions have no right or wrong responses. The following list gives some examples of ethical issues of reproduction.

- The *Roe v. Wade* abortion decision is challenged before the U.S. Supreme Court.
- Surrogate parenting is now illegal in several states.
- A grandmother in South Africa gives birth to her own grandchild (conceived through in vitro fertilization).
- Against the wishes of relatives, an Australian judge ordered frozen embryos to be implanted in a surrogate after the millionaire parents were killed in a plane crash.
- A daughter becomes pregnant in order to donate aborted fetal tissues to help her father combat Parkinson's disease.
- A man sues his ex-wife to prevent implantation of frozen embryos after divorce.
- Selective abortion to choose gender and other genetic characteristics is now possible in cases of multiple pregnancies (e.g., twins, triplets, and so forth).
- Hundreds of babies born to drug-addicted mothers live in hospitals as boarder babies.
- One baby with a birth defect is allowed to die, but another with the same condition is given lifesaving surgery; the hospital's decision is based on the family's economic ability to care for a disabled child.
- A surgeon provides free surgery to infertile women living on welfare to make conception possible.

Examining the Evidence

1. The ethical issues surrounding reproductive function find people on both sides of the dispute. Why do you think that coming to an agreement as to what is "right" or "wrong" in these situations is so difficult?

   _____

   _____

   _____

2. Which interested parties do you think should be on an ethical committee of a hospital or health care agency to determine the course of action in these situations?

   _____

   _____

   _____

3. What factors do you think are most important in making ethical decisions about these issues (e.g., economic, social, religious, legal)? Explain the reasoning that supports your position.

   _____

   _____

   _____

4. List the three issues that concern you the most of those presented earlier or that currently are in the news.

   _____

   _____

   _____

5. Explain your position on one of the three issues you listed in question 4.

   _____

   _____

   _____

6. Why might someone have a view that differs from the one you stated in question 5?

_____

_____

_____

INTERNET ACTIVITIES

Reproductive System Topics

Use the Internet to research one of the following topics related to the sensory system. Write an essay, make a poster, or make a pamphlet that describes the topic.

Sexually Transmitted Infections
Suggested Website

KidsHealth: http://kidshealth.org/teen/sexual_health/stds/std.html

Teenage Pregnancy
Suggested Websites

March of Dimes: http://www.marchofdimes.com/professionals/14332_1159.asp
CDC: http://www.cdc.gov/reproductivehealth/AdolescentReproHealth/index.htm

Essay

_____

_____

_____

_____

_____

_____

_____

_____

_____

_____

_____

_____

_____

_____

_____

_____

_____

_____

_____

_____

_____

_____

238

22 Laboratory Careers

Complete the crossword puzzle using the Key Terms.

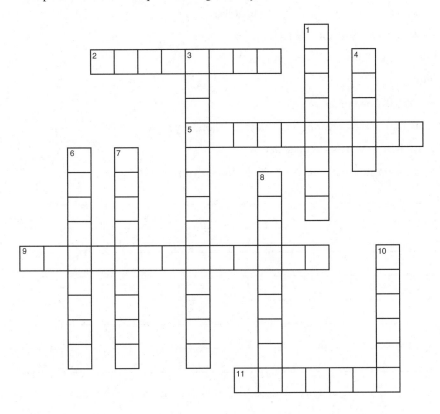

ACROSS

2 High level of resistance to certain microorganisms or diseases
5 Incision into a vein to withdraw blood
9 Microscopic living organism, microbe
11 Free from all living microorganisms

DOWN

1 Microorganism that produces disease
3 Microorganism that does not produce disease
4 Person who supplies living tissue or who furnishes blood or blood products for transfusion to another person
6 Invasion and multiplication of pathogenic microorganisms in the body tissues
7 Cell that surrounds and destroys microorganisms and foreign particles
8 One who receives tissue from another, such as in a blood transfusion
10 Inanimate object capable of carrying germs

ABBREVIATIONS

Match each of the following abbreviations with the phrase that best describes its meaning or function. Then write the phrase or name for each of the abbreviations in the spaces provided.

Abbreviation

1. _____ CBC
2. _____ CLS
3. _____ CT
4. _____ ESR
5. _____ Hct
6. _____ Hgb
7. _____ MD
8. _____ MLA
9. _____ MLT
10. _____ MT

Meaning or Function

a. Blood bank specialist

b. CLS that passes Registry testing

c. Lab workers who may specialize in histology

d. Lab workers who perform phlebotomy

e. Molecule that carries oxygen in the cells

f. Pathologist

g. Rate of RBC precipitation

h. Technologist who performs and analyzes laboratory tests

i. Test for RBCs, WBCs, and platelets

j. Test that measures the percent of whole blood that is RBCs

1. CBC: _____

2. CLS: _____

3. CT: _____

4. ESR: _____

5. Hct: _____

6. Hgb: _____

7. MD: _____

8. MLA: _____

9. MLT: _____

10. MT: _____

JUST THE FACTS

1. The _ _ ⊙ _ _ _ _ _ _ _ _ is a medical doctor who examines specimens of body tissue, fluids, and secretions to diagnose disease.

2. Areas of specialization for a laboratory technologist include _ _ _ _ _ _ _ _ _ _ _ _ _ _, chemistry, _ _ _ _ _ _ _ _ _ _, and immunology.

3. Microbiologists study _ _ _ _ ⊙ _ _ _, _ _ _ _ _ _ _, _ _ _ _ _ _ _ _, and other microorganisms that cause disease or may be used to prevent it.

4. Some microorganisms are always present (_ _ _ _ _ _ _ ⊙), and some are found temporarily (_ _ _ _ _ _ _ _ _ _).

5. _ _ _ _ _ _ _ _ _ is a state of disease caused by the presence of pathogenic microorganisms in the body.

6. Four groups of microorganisms that cause disease in humans are _ _ _ _ _ _ _ _ _, fungi,

_ _ _ _ _ _ _ _ Ⓞ _ _, and viruses.

7. _ _ _ _ _ _ _ _ _ _ _ _ _ is the study of diseases occurring in human populations.

8. _ _ _ Ⓞ _ _ _ _ _ _ _ is the study of how the blood cells prevent disease caused by

microorganisms.

9. The first line of defense is the _ _ _ Ⓞ, a second defense is the action of

_ _ _ _ _ _ _ _ _ _ _ cells.

10. One of the skills used by laboratory personnel is the preparation of bacterial cultures using

Ⓞ _ _ _ _ _ _ technique.

Use the circled letters to form the answer to this jumble. Clue: What is a bacterial infection that may result from a puncture wound?

_ _ _ _ _ _ _

CONCEPT APPLICATIONS

Identifying Disease-Causing Microorganisms

Use Table 22-5 of the textbook and the Internet to label the diagrams of microorganisms in Figure 22-1, A to F. In the spaces provided in Table 22-1, list two diseases that each of the types of organism causes in humans.

A _____   B 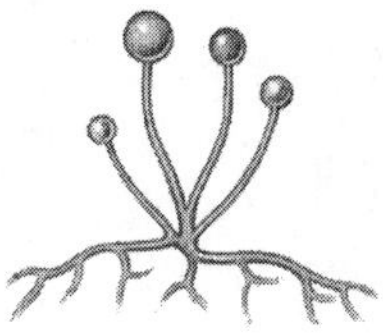 _____   C _____

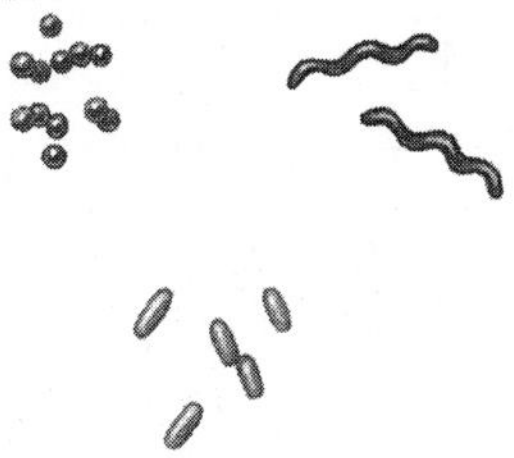

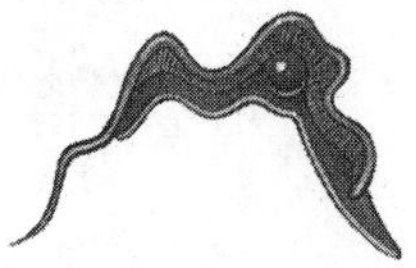

D _____   E _____   F _____

Figure 22-1

Chapter **22** **Laboratory Careers**

TABLE 22-1 Disease-Causing Microorganisms

ORGANISM	EXAMPLES
Bacteria	
Metazoan	
Mold	
Protozoan	
Virus	
Yeast	

Identifying Parts of the Microscope

Use Figure 22-12 of the textbook to label the parts of the microscope in Figure 22-2.

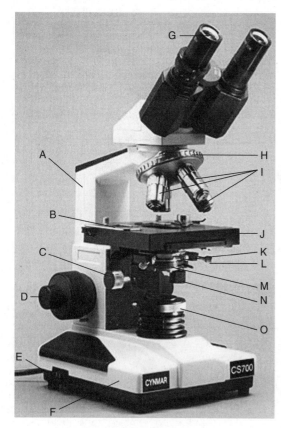

Figure 22-2

A. _____

B. _____

C. _____

D. _____

E. _____

F. _____

G. _____

H. _____

I. _____

J. _____

K. _____

L. _____

M. _____

N. _____

O. _____

Laboratory Careers

Laboratory Skills and Qualities

List three personal qualities and skills that are important in laboratory careers.

1. _____

2. _____

3. _____

Identifying Laboratory Careers

Use the textbook to provide the missing information about laboratory careers in Table 22-2.

TABLE 22-2 Laboratory Careers

CAREER TITLE	YEARS OF EDUCATION	DESCRIPTION OF JOB DUTIES	CREDENTIALS REQUIRED
			BS, some states require licensure
		Preparation of tissue slides, analysis of blood samples, urinalysis under supervision	
		Development of new drugs and plant varieties, environmental protection	
Food scientist			
		Makes prostheses, including bridges, denture, and crowns	

Applying Your Knowledge

1. The medical doctor who often manages the laboratory and examines body tissues and fluids is called a

   _____.

2. The _____ would examine urine to assist in diagnosing a bladder infection.

3. The professional who would be involved in the research and study of HIV is probably a

   _____.

4. The study of body specimens to determine hormonal and chemical changes at the cellular level is performed by a

   technologist specializing in _____.

5. Safe food processing is evaluated by the _____.

INVESTIGATIONS

Using the Microscope to Identify Microorganisms

Review the directions for use of the microscope found in the textbook in Skill List 22-4. You will be assigned a microorganism or secretion specimen by your teacher. Read all of the directions before beginning this activity. Laboratory activities should be completed under the supervision of a qualified professional only.

Equipment and Supplies

Cover slip
Eyedropper
Microscope
Microscope slide
Prepared slide of microorganism
Unknown specimen
Water

Directions

1. Maintain medical asepsis by practicing good handwashing technique.
2. Follow the directions for microscope use to observe and draw the prepared slide under low, medium, and high power in Figure 22-3.

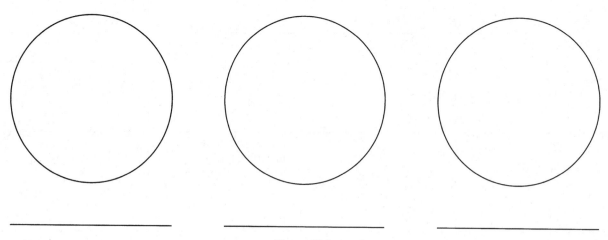

Figure 22-3

3. Prepare a wet mount slide by placing a small amount of the unknown specimen in the center of a clean slide. Add a drop of water to the specimen if it is not already in a solution.
4. Cover the specimen with a clean cover slip.
5. Follow the directions for microscope use to observe and draw the prepared slide under low, medium, and high power in Figure 22-4.
6. Clean and return all materials to the designated location.

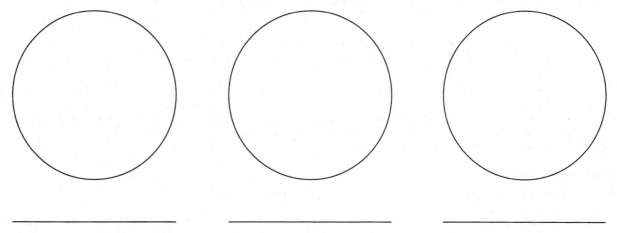

Figure 22-4

Drawing Conclusions

1. How does the field of vision, or amount of the specimen, compare when the microscope is switched from low to high power?

_____

_____

_____

2. Why is it important to look at the objective from the side when moving it toward the stage?

_____

_____

_____

3. What does *parfocal* mean?

_____

_____

_____

Identifying Microorganisms in the School and Home Environment

Review the information in the textbook regarding preparation of sterile agar plates and transfer of bacteria before beginning this activity. Many bacteria can be found in common household and school environments. Read all of the directions before beginning this activity. Laboratory activities should be completed under the supervision of a qualified professional only.

Equipment and Supplies

Autoclave or bleach
Grease pencil or china marker
Incubator
Sterile culture swab
Sterile nutrient agar plate

Directions

1. Maintain medical asepsis by practicing good handwashing technique.
2. Prepare a sterile agar plate and culture swab. A wooden cotton swab can be sterilized for use as a culture swab.
3. Collect a specimen by rubbing the cotton swab on a surface in your environment. Do not allow the cotton swab to touch any other surface.
4. Open the sterile plate to inoculate the agar with the culture swab. Close the plate immediately.
5. Discard the culture swab in the proper receptacle.
6. Mark the bottom of a sterile agar plate with the site of specimen collection, date, and your initials.
7. Place the closed plate in an incubator at 37° C. Place the plate upside down to prevent condensation or liquid from forming on the specimen.
8. Incubate the plate for 3 or 4 days. Make observations for each 24-hour period.
9. Count the number of different types of bacterial colonies on the plate. Create a data chart or drawing to record your results.
10. Compare your results with other locations in the environment.
11. To prevent the spread of unknown microorganisms, sterilize or disinfect the agar before discarding it.
12. You may repeat the procedure by testing for airborne microorganisms only. For this activity, the plate should be exposed to the air in different locations for a designated length of time before incubation.
13. Clean and return all materials to the designated location.

Drawing Conclusions

1. How many and what type of bacterial colonies did your plate show after incubation?

_____

_____

_____

2. In what area of the environment did your class find the most bacterial growth?

_____

_____

_____

3. Why is it important to sterilize or disinfect the culture plates before discarding them?

_____

_____

_____

4. Why is 37° C used for incubation of the microorganisms?

_____

_____

_____

5. Why were the bacteria not visible before incubation?

_____

_____

_____

Demonstrating the Effect of Antibiotics on Bacteria

Antibiotics are chemical substances that kill microorganisms or inhibit their growth. Most antibiotics are made from natural waste products of fungi and bacteria. Antibiotics have varied levels of effectiveness in killing different bacteria. Before an antibiotic is prescribed, it is helpful to know which one would be most effective. The following activity determines which antibiotic is most effective in inhibiting the growth of known bacteria.

Chapter **22** *Laboratory Careers*

Antibiotic-resistant types of bacteria are common in hospitals because so many antibiotics are used in those facilities.

Before beginning this activity, review the information in the textbook about the correct way to transfer bacteria. Nonpathogenic bacteria and antibiotic dots may be purchased for this activity from a biological supply service.

Read all of the directions before beginning this activity. Laboratory activities should be completed under the supervision of a qualified professional only.

Equipment and Supplies

Antibiotic disks
Autoclave or bleach
China marker
Incubator
Known nonpathogenic bacteria
Sterile culture swab or inoculating loop
Sterile forceps or antibiotic disk dispenser
Sterile nutrient agar plate

Directions

1. Maintain medical asepsis by practicing good handwashing technique.
2. Use sterile technique to transfer the known nonpathogenic bacteria from the culture tube to a sterile nutrient agar plate. Streak the surface evenly without breaking the surface of the agar.
3. Use a sterile forceps or antibiotic dispenser to space three or four different antibiotic dots evenly on the surface of the agar.
4. Use a china marker to label each section of the agar plate on the bottom of the plate; note the date, your initials, and the types of antibiotics used.
5. Place the Petri dish upside down in an incubator at 37° C for 3 or 4 days.
6. Observe the agar plate for clear areas around each antibiotic disk. The halo, or zone of inhibition, indicates that the antibiotic inhibited the growth of the bacteria in that area. The size of the zone indicates how effective the antibiotic is in stopping bacterial growth.
7. Measure the width of each zone of inhibition. Record the results in Table 22-3.
8. Sterilize or disinfect the cultures before discarding them.
9. Clean and return all materials to the designated location.

TABLE 22-3 Effect of Antibiotics on Bacteria

Type of microorganism:			
Type of antibiotic		Size of halo	
Type of antibiotic		Size of halo	
Type of antibiotic		Size of halo	
Type of antibiotic		Size of halo	

Drawing Conclusions

1. Which antibiotic was most effective against the bacteria?

_____

_____

_____

2. What are four items necessary for the growth of bacterial colonies?

_____

_____

_____

3. What are two precautions that you used during the activity to protect yourself and the agar medium from contamination with unknown microorganisms?

_____

_____

_____

4. What are two potential sources of error in your activity?

_____

_____

_____

Demonstrating the Effect of Disinfectants on Bacteria

Review the information in the textbook on the correct method of transferring bacteria before beginning this activity. Disinfectants are chemical compounds that inhibit the growth of microorganisms. Nonpathogenic bacteria may be purchased for this activity from a biological supply service.

Read all of the directions before beginning this activity. Laboratory activities should be completed under the supervision of a qualified professional only.

Equipment and Supplies

Autoclave or bleach
Disinfectants
Incubator
Nonpathogenic bacteria
Sterile forceps
Sterile nutrient agar plate
Sterile swab or inoculating loop
Sterile filter disks soaked with disinfectants

Directions

1. Maintain medical asepsis by practicing good handwashing technique.
2. Transfer the known nonpathogenic bacteria from the culture tube to a sterile agar plate. Streak the agar evenly without breaking the surface.
3. Dip a small, sterile filter disk into a household disinfectant.
4. Use sterile forceps to space three or four different disinfectant filter dots evenly on the surface of the agar.
5. Use a china marker to label each section on the bottom of the agar plate; note the date, your initials, and the types of disinfectants used.
6. Place the Petri dish upside down in an incubator at 37° C for 3 or 4 days.
7. Observe the agar plate for clear areas around each disinfectant disk. The halo, or zone of inhibition, indicates that the disinfectant inhibited the growth of the bacteria in that area. The size of the halo indicates the effectiveness of the disinfectant in stopping bacterial growth.
8. Measure the width of each zone of inhibition. Record the results in Table 22-4.
9. Sterilize or disinfect the cultures before discarding them.
10. Clean and return all materials to the designated location.

TABLE 22-4 Effect of Disinfectants on Bacteria

Type of microorganism:			
Type of antibiotic		Size of halo	
Type of antibiotic		Size of halo	
Type of antibiotic		Size of halo	
Type of antibiotic		Size of halo	

Drawing Conclusions

1. Which disinfectant was most effective against the bacteria?

_____

_____

_____

2. What are two precautions that you used during the activity to protect yourself and the agar medium from contamination with unknown microorganisms?

_____

_____

_____

3. What are two sources of error in your activity?

_____

_____

_____

4. What is the difference between a disinfectant and an antibiotic?

_____

_____

_____

CRITICAL THINKING

Laboratory Safety

No set of policies and procedures can cover all of the situations in which hazards in the medical laboratory might occur. However, practicing some simple rules and using common sense can make the laboratory a safe environment. The following are some of the rules of safety that apply to any laboratory environment.

Laboratory Safety Guidelines

1. Read all instructions about any unfamiliar procedure before attempting it.
2. Do not eat, drink, smoke, or chew gum in the laboratory area. Do not place supplies, equipment, or chemicals in the mouth.
3. Keep the laboratory area clean and free of debris. Store equipment and supplies in the designated manner and location after use.
4. Wear gloves when handling body secretions and at all times if open sores or cuts are present on the hands. Wash hands frequently and when any laboratory chemical or specimen is accidentally touched.
5. Handle all laboratory equipment with care, and follow the manufacturer's instructions at all times.
6. Report damaged equipment and supplies promptly. Clean any spills or breakage promptly and in an appropriate manner.
7. Do not replace used chemicals into stock bottles. Handle chemicals, test tubes, and other supplies and equipment with the appropriate utensil.
8. Wear safety glasses and masks as needed when handling toxic chemicals and when running the autoclave.
9. Do not wear jewelry or clothing that hangs loose or dangles. Confine hair in a band or net to keep it away from the face and neck. Wear a standard laboratory jacket and closed-toed shoes.
10. Avoid horseplay and other dangerous behaviors at all times. Report any accident or injury to the supervisor immediately.
11. Keep visitors and non-laboratory personnel in a designated area away from the laboratory work.
12. Know the location of and how to use diagnostic and laboratory equipment, including a fire extinguisher, fire blanket, and laboratory shower.

Examining the Evidence

1. What does the term *common sense* mean?

_____

_____

_____

2. Explain the importance of five of the safety guidelines.

   (1) _____

   _____

   _____

   (2) _____

   _____

   _____

   (3) _____

   _____

   _____

   (4) _____

   _____

   _____

   (5) _____

   _____

   _____

3. For what other reason, in addition to safety, would it be important to follow the guidelines?

_____

_____

_____

4. Which individual in the laboratory is most responsible for laboratory safety?

_____

_____

_____

Education and Career Research

Use the following links, other Internet resources, and information available by telephone or mail inquiry to determine the educational cost of one laboratory career and the salary that might be earned in the local area. Use the information to complete Table 22-5.

Suggested Websites

Salary.com: http://salary.com
Monster.com: http://monster.com
Occupational Outlook Handbook: http://www.bls.gov/oco/
American Society for Clinical Laboratory Science: http://www.ascls.org/

TABLE 22-5 Education and Career Research

CAREER	INSTITUTION FOR EDUCATION	COST OF EDUCATION	POTENTIAL EARNINGS

VAPID VOCABULARY

Complete the crossword puzzle using the Key Terms.

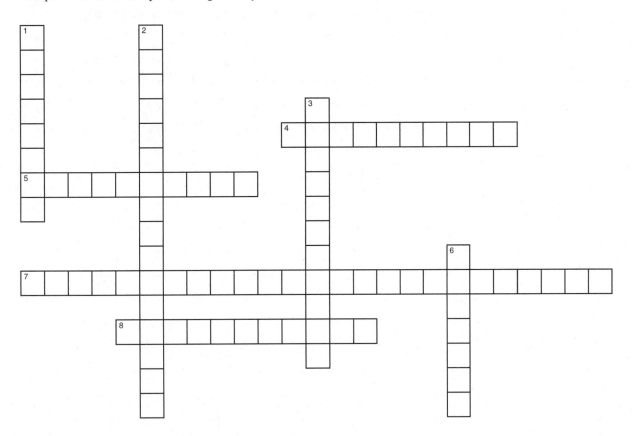

ACROSS

4 Visualization of deep structures of the body by recording reflections of sound waves directed into the tissues

5 Radiograph producing a detailed cross section of tissue at a predetermined depth

7 A chemical that does not permit passage of x-rays (three words)

8 Making film records of internal structures by passing radiographs or gamma rays through the body to make images on specially sensitized film; roentgenography

DOWN

1 Distinction between positive and negative charges of particles

2 Recording the position and motion of the heart walls or its internal structures using ultrasonic waves

3 Immediate visualization of part of the body on a screen using radiography

6 One or more forms of an atom with a difference in the number of neutrons

ABBREVIATIONS

Match each of the following abbreviations with the phrase that best describes its meaning or function. Then write the phrase or name for each of the abbreviations in the spaces provided.

Abbreviation	Meaning or Function
1. _____ CT	a. Detailed image produced using a magnetic field
2. _____ DR	b. First technique used to link computers to radiographs
3. _____ DX	c. Misleading term for procedure that does not use radioactive materials
4. _____ ECHO	d. Noninvasive measuring of cerebral functions
5. _____ MRI	e. One of two abbreviations used for a technique that does not use film
6. _____ NIR	f. One of two abbreviations used for a technique that does not use film
7. _____ NMRI	g. Technologist that injects radioisotopes for basic and emergency care
8. _____ NMT	h. Two dimensional images produced using sound waves
9. _____ PET	i. Ultrasounds used to visualize the heart and blood vessels
10. _____ SONO	j. Visualizes metabolic activities of the body

1. CT: _____

2. DR: _____

3. DX: _____

4. ECHO: _____

5. MRI: _____

6. NIR: _____

7. NMRI: _____

8. NMT: _____

9. PET: _____

10. SONO: _____

JUST THE FACTS

1. Radiology technologists work under the direction of a ○ _ _ _ _ _ _ _ _ and may specialize in one area of diagnosis or treatment.

2. Radiology work includes some hazard of radiation exposure, so each worker wears a _ _ _ _ _ _ _ _ _ that records the level of exposure to radiological materials.

3. Radioactive compounds may be _ _ _ _ _ ○ _ _ into the bloodstream, _ _ _ _ _ ○ _ _ _, or _ _ _ _ _ _ _ _.

4. _ _ _ _ _ _ _ _ _ _ _ _ _ _ _ _ _ _ technicians may work in the radiology department or area and monitor or test the action of the heart.

5. _ ○ _ technologists measure the electrical activity of the brain.

6. The field of radiography has expanded greatly as modern methods of imaging have combined the use of

_ _ _ _ _ _ _ _ _ _ with radiographic procedures.

7. _ _ _ _ _ _Ⓞ_ _ _ _ _ _ _ _ _ _ _ tomography uses computers and radio-

graphic technique to visualize the metabolic activities of the body as well as its structure.

8. _ _ _ _ _ _ _Ⓞ_ _ _ _ _ _ _ _ _ _ imaging is a process that creates

superb image resolution and tissue contrast.

9. A _ Ⓞ _ _ _ _ _ _ _ is a radiograph of the breast used to detect cancer.

10. Near infrared _ _ _ _ _ _ _ _ _ _ _ _ _ Ⓞ is a technique that allows

_ _ _ _ _ _ _ _ _ _ _ measuring of cerebral functions.

Use the circled letters to form the answer to this jumble. Clue: What is the property of cells that allows radiologists to use magnets to produce images?

_ _ _ _ _ _ _ _ _

CONCEPT APPLICATIONS

Imaging Careers
Imaging Skills and Qualities
List three personal qualities and skills that are important in imaging careers.

1. _____

2. _____

3. _____

Identifying Imaging Careers

Use the textbook to provide the missing information about imaging careers in Table 23-1.

TABLE 23-1 Imaging Careers

CAREER TITLE	YEARS OF EDUCATION	DESCRIPTION OF JOB DUTIES AND OPPORTUNITIES	CREDENTIALS
		Produce two-dimensional images of internal organs using sound waves at high frequency	
		Transfer and position the patient, select materials for making images, including radiopaque	
		Use computers and magnets to produce an image of the internal soft tissues	
		Prepare and administer radioactive compounds	
	On-the-job or 1- to 2-year program		

Applying Your Knowledge

1. The imaging health care worker who might be found in the emergency department to assist with the diagnosis of a

   broken arm would be the _____.

2. An _____ performs tests that may help determine fetal age.

3. A brain tumor might be diagnosed using the radioactive tests performed by the

   _____.

4. The health care worker who may assist with diagnosing abnormal electrical activity of the brain is the

   _____.

5. The _____ would administer the radiation treatment for many types of cancer.

256

INVESTIGATIONS

Determining the Effect of Light Rays

Light and radiographic waves come from the same electromagnetic spectrum and share many of the same properties. Work in groups of two or three for this activity. Read all of the directions before beginning the activity. Laboratory activities should be completed under the supervision of a qualified professional only.

Equipment and Supplies

Construction paper (optional)
Flashlight
Penlight
Yardstick

Directions

1. Hold a flashlight perpendicular to the wall at a distance of 1 foot.
2. Measure the diameter of the image produced by the beam on the wall.
3. Repeat the procedure, holding the flashlight 2, 3, 4, and 5 feet from the wall. Record the results in Table 23-2.
4. Repeat steps 1 through 3, using the penlight as the energy source. Record the results in Table 23-2.
5. Using the flashlight as the energy source, repeat steps 1 through 3 while holding a piece of construction paper 6 inches from the wall between the wall and beam of the flashlight during all measurements. Record the results in Table 23-2.

TABLE 23-2 Effect of Light Rays

DISTANCE	1 FOOT	2 FEET	3 FEET	4 FEET	5 FEET
Flashlight					
Penlight					
Construction paper					

Drawing Conclusions

1. How does the area covered by the beam from the light source that is near the wall compare with the area covered at a greater distance?

_____

_____

_____

2. Was the beam produced by the light source stronger or weaker in intensity as it was moved farther from the wall?

_____

_____

_____

3. Why does the operator of radiographic equipment maintain as great a distance from the beam as possible?

_____

_____

_____

4. How does the construction paper placed between the light source and wall represent the action of a lead shield used in radiography?

_____

_____

_____

Calculating the Intensity of Energy Sources

Beams of energy follow the law of intensity called the *inverse square law of radiation*. It states that the intensity of the radiation beam is inversely proportional to the square of the distance from the source.

Examining the Evidence

1. Use Table 23-2 to calculate the intensity of the light produced by the flashlight from the distances measured. What are these values?

_____

_____

_____

2. Does the inverse square law apply to the beam produced by the light source?

_____

_____

_____

INTERNET ACTIVITIES

Education and Career Research

Use the following links, other Internet resources, and information available by telephone or mail inquiry to determine the educational cost of one imaging career and the salary that might be earned in the local area. Use the information to complete Table 23-3.

Suggested Websites

Salary.com: http://salary.com
Monster.com: http://monster.com
Occupational Outlook Handbook: http://www.bls.gov/oco/
Radiology Info: http://www.radiologyinfo.org/

TABLE 23-3 Education and Career Research

CAREER	INSTITUTION FOR EDUCATION	COST OF EDUCATION	POTENTIAL EARNINGS

VAPID VOCABULARY

Complete the crossword puzzle using the Key Terms.

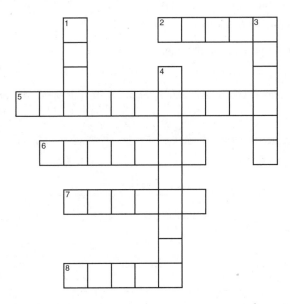

ACROSS

2 Heartbeat that can be felt, or palpated, on surface arteries as the artery walls expand with blood
5 Within a vein or veins
6 Process of removing pathogenic microorganisms or protecting against infection by such organisms
7 Pertaining to, or located at, the apex of the heart
8 Necessary to life

DOWN

1 Part of a facility, including equipment and supplies organized to provide specific care
3 Vomit
4 Pertaining to the period shortly before and after birth

ABBREVIATIONS

Match each of the following abbreviations with the phrase that best describes its meaning or function. Then write the phrase or name for each of the abbreviations in the spaces provided.

Abbreviation

1. _____ ADL
2. _____ ADPIE
3. _____ ANA
4. _____ BLS
5. _____ BSN
6. _____ CNA
7. _____ HS (hs)
8. _____ LPN
9. _____ RN
10. _____ ROM

Meaning or Function

a. Basic care
b. Evening
c. Four-year program in nursing
d. Government information and statistics on jobs
e. Minimum 150 training program in nursing
f. Movement to prevent contractures
g. Nurse who has been approved by the state after three- or four-year program
h. Nursing process
i. Organization, also called *Nursing World*
j. Three-year program in nursing

1. ADL: _____

2. ADPIE: _____

3. ANA: _____

4. BLS: _____

5. BSN: _____

6. CNA: _____

7. HS (hs): _____

8. LPN: _____

9. RN: _____

10. ROM: _____

JUST THE FACTS

1. Registered _ _ ◯ _ _ ◯ make up the largest group of health care workers, with more than 2 million jobs.

2. The function of the nurse is to promote _ _ _ _ _ _ _ health and _ _ _ _ _ ◯ _ care during illness.

3. Three levels of nursing care include the _ _ _ _ _ _ _ _ _ _ nurse, ◯ _ _ _ _ _ _ _ _   _ _ _ _ _ ◯ _ _ _ nurse, and nursing _ _ _ _ _ _ _ _ _.

4. Advanced preparation by the registered nurse may lead to work as a nurse _ _ _ _ _ _ _ _ _ _ _ _ _, clinical nurse _ _ _ _ _ _ _ _ _ _, nurse _ _ _ _ _ _ _ _ _ _ _ _, or nurse _ _ _ _ _ ◯ _.

5. Areas of specialization for the _ ◯ _ _ _ _ _ _ _, nurse include units, such as the operating room, recovery room, critical care, and emergency room.

6. Nursing assistants may provide care in the patient's home and are called _ _ _ _ Ⓞ _ _ _ assistants.

7. Within a 24-hour period, the fluid that is taken into the body and eliminated from the body should be approximately equal in volume to maintain the balance of the _ _ _ _ _ _ _ _ _ _ _ _ _ and Ⓠ _ _ _ _ needed to perform body processes.

8. Oral intake is considered to be anything that is _ _ _ Ⓞ _ _ at room temperature and taken by _ _ _ _ _.

9. _ _ _ _ _ _ _ _ _ _ _ _ _ exercises are designed to move the muscles and tendons of the joints for patients who are not able to move independently or have limited abilities.

10. Maintaining an orderly and safe environment for care of the patient is the responsibility of _ _ _ health care _ _ _ _ _ _ _ _ _ _ Ⓞ _ _ _ _.

Use the circled letters to form the answer to this jumble. Clue: What is the phrase used when the patient is offered at least 100 mL of liquid every hour?

_ _ _ _ _ _ _ _ _ _ _

CONCEPT APPLICATIONS

Recording Daily Care
Review the information provided in Chapter 2 and Chapter 7 regarding assessment and recording of vital signs.

Use the information provided in Figure 24-1, Mrs. Jewel's hospital stay graphic sheet, to complete the care flow sheet in Figure 24-2.

Drawing Conclusions
1. How well did Mrs. Jewel eat breakfast and lunch on the day recorded?

_____

_____

_____

2. Why did the health care assistant omit the dinner meal?

_____

_____

_____

3. What is the level of responsiveness and orientation of Mrs. Jewel?

_____

_____

_____

Jewel, Martha
Nelson, Douglas, M.D.
Room 506
Appendicitis

GRAPHIC RECORD
SIDE A

DATE	1-15-10	1-16-10	1-17-10	1-18-10	1-19-10
HOSPITAL DAYS	-Admit-	-2-	-3-	-4-	-5-
P.O. DAY	–	–	-1-	-2-	

	AM			PM			AM			PM			AM			PM			AM			PM			AM			PM		
HOUR	4	8	12	4	8	12	4	8	12	4	8	12	4	8	12	4	8	12	4	8	12	4	8	12	4	8	12	4	8	12

TEMPERATURE scale: C 40°/39°/38°/37°/36° — F 104°/103°/102°/101°/100°/99°/98.6°/98°/97°/96°

(Temperature plotted: ~101° at PM 8 on 1-15-10 declining to ~99° by 1-15-10 PM 12; "To Surgery" noted on 1-16-10; temperatures around 98.6°–99° on 1-17-10 and 1-18-10; "Discharged" noted on 1-18-10/1-19-10)

PULSE				88	84	76																								
RESPIRATION				20	18	16																								
BLOOD PRESSURE				134/84	130/80	124/74																								

HEIGHT	WT. 125 lb.	WT.	WT.	WT.	WT.
24 HR. TOTAL INTAKE	500 cc+	Parenteral-900 cc 100 cc+	850 cc	650 cc	
24 HR. TOTAL OUTPUT	700 cc+	850 cc	780 cc	700 cc	
STOOL				ꭲ Formed, Brown	
STOOL FOR GUAIAC	—	—	—	—	—

Figure 24-1

CARE FLOW SHEET

CLIENT NAME : __Jewel, Martha_____ _____   ROOM NO. : ___506_____

	7–3	3–11	11–7
Bath/Shower/Bedbath	Shower 9:00 _SS_		
Hair Care	9:15 _SS_		
Back Rub/Skin Care	9:15 _SS_		
Nails	——		
Shave	——		
Oral Hygiene	Self 8:00 _SS_		
Temperature			
Pulse			
Respiration			
Blood Pressure			
Urine Output			
Bowel Movement			
Level of Consciousness	Alert _SS_		
Orientation	Oriented × 3 _SS_		
Breakfast (% Eaten)	80%		
Lunch (% Eaten)	50%		
Dinner (% Eaten)	——		
Clinitest	——		
Acetest	——		
Sleep/Rest	——		
Specimen	——		
Other	——		

SIGNATURE : _SSmith_ ————   TITLE : _LPN_ ————   DATE : _1-18-10_____

SIGNATURE : _____   TITLE : _____   DATE : _____

SIGNATURE : _____   TITLE : _____   DATE : _____

Figure 24-2

Assessing Tissue Integrity and Safety Needs

Study the tissue integrity survey in Figure 24-3 and the safety assessment in Figure 24-4 for Mrs. Jewel during her hospital stay.

Jewel, Martha
Nelson, Douglas, M.D.
Room 506
Appendicitis

ASSESSMENT FORM
- TISSUE INTEGRITY
- PATIENT SAFETY

TISSUE INTEGRITY ASSESSMENT FORM

Identify any patient at risk of developing pressure sores. Assess the seven clinical condition parameters to determine a patient risk score. Patients with a score of twelve or more should be considered at risk of developing pressure sores. Initiate preventive protocol per patient care plan.

CLINICAL CONDITION PARAMETERS	adm.	72hrs.	1wk.
GENERAL PHYSICAL CONDITION (health problems) Good(minor) ....0 Fair (acute/chronic - but stable) ....1 Poor (acute/chronic - not stable) ....2 Terminal 3	0	0	
LEVEL OF CONSCIOUSNESS (to commands) Alert (responds readily) ....0 Lethargic (slow to respond) ....1 Semi-comatose or Confused................2 (responds only to painful/verbal stimuli) Comatose (no response to stimuli) 3	0	0	
ACTIVITY Ambulatory without assistance ....0 Ambulatory with assistance ....2 Chair and/or bed only ....4 Confined to bed................6	2	2	
MOBILITY - RANGE OF MOTION Full active range of motion ....0 Moves with limited assistance ....2 Moves only with assistance................4 Immobile................6	2	2	
GENERAL SKIN CONDITION Healthy (clean, clear, supple) ....0 Fair (rashes or abrasions)................2 Poor (dry, poor tugor, advanced age) ....6 Edema, reddened areas, "thin skin" ....8 Pressure sore (document on Flowsheet)... 12	0	0	
INCONTINENCE (bowel and/or bladder) None ....0 Foley catheter ....1 Occasional (<3 per 24hr) ....2 Usually (>3 per 24hr) ....4 Total (no control) 6	0	0	
NUTRITION (for age and size) Good (eats/drinks 75-100% of meals) ....0 Fair (eats/drinks 50-75% of meals) ....1 Tube Feeding/Hyperalimentation ....2 Poor (unable or refuses to eat or drink) 3	1	0	
TOTAL SCORE	5	4	

	Date	Init.	Signature
Adm.	1-15-10	*S.S.*	*S. Smith, LPN*
72hrs.	1-17-10	*S.S.*	*S. Smith, LPN*
1wk.			

Figure 24-3

Jewel, Martha
Nelson, Douglas, M.D.
Room 506
Appendicitis

PATIENT SAFETY ASSESSMENT FORM

Identify any patient at risk for fall by assessing the 11 parameters listed and assigning a score (0=least risk and 5=greatest risk). Patients with a score of 15 or above should be considered at risk for a fall and a care plan with appropriate nursing intervention should be developed.

CLINICAL PARAMETERS		adm.	72hrs.	1wk.
1. Unsteady on feet		2	4	
2. Poor eyesight (glasses=1)		1	1	
3. Changes in environment		1	3	
4. Drugs or alcohol		0	0	
5. Physical disabilities		0	0	
6. Multiple diagnosis		0	0	
7. Language barrier		0	0	
8. Neurological problems		0	0	
9. Attitude		1	2	
10. Confused & disoriented	15pts.	0	0	
11. Previous fall	15pts.	0	0	
TOTAL SCORE		4	10	

	Date	Init.	Signature
Adm.	1-15-10	S. S.	S. Smith L P N
72hrs.	1-17-10	S. S.	S. Smith L P N
1wk.			

Figure 24-4

Drawing Conclusions

1. How did the safety assessment change during the first 72 hours of Mrs. Jewel's stay in the hospital?

_____

_____

_____

2. What might have caused the change in the risk factors considered in this assessment?

_____

_____

_____

Temperature Conversion and Charting Vital Signs

Convert the temperature readings in the last column of the following table, and use the information to chart the following vital signs in Figures 24-5 and 24-6.

DATE	TIME	VITAL SIGNS			
9/1	8:00 AM	BP 124/98	P 76	R 20	T 98.6° F orally
	12:00 PM	BP 122/76	P 78	R 16	T 98.2° F orally
	4:00 PM	BP 120/82	P 70	R 18	T 99.0° F orally
	8:00 PM	BP 118/76	P 64	R 22	T 102.0° F rectally
9/2	12:00 AM	BP 124/78	P 80	R 26	T 104.2° F rectally
	8:00 AM	BP 116/76	P 68	R 16	T 98.2° F orally
	4:00 PM	BP 122/82	P 72	R 20	T 98.6° F orally
9/3	8:00 AM	BP 120/76	P 68	R 16	T 98.2° F orally
	4:00 PM	BP 126/98	P 74	R 14	T 98.6° F orally

GRAPHIC RECORD

	DATE																								

	HOUR	2400	0400	0800	1200	1600	2000	2400	0400	0800	1200	1600	2000	2400	0400	0800	1200	1600	2000	2400	0400	0800	1200	1600	2000

TEMPERATURE

42.
41.5
41.
40.5
40.
39.5
39.
38.5
38.
37.5
37.
36.5
36.

PULSE																								

RESPIRATION																								

	TIME				
BLOOD PRESSURE	2400				
	0400				
	0800				
	1200				
	1600				
	2000				

Figure 24-5

GRAPHIC CHART (Fahrenheit)

Date																															
Hospital Days																															
Day P.O. or P.P																															
HOUR		0400	0800	1200	1600	2000	2400	0400	0800	1200	1600	2000	2400	0400	0800	1200	1600	2000	2400	0400	0800	1200	1600	2000	2400	0400	0800	1200	1600	2000	2400

PULSE (Red) / TEMPERATURE (Black)

	F
150	106°
140	105°
130	104°
120	103°
110	102°
100	101°
90	100°
80	99°
	98.6°
70	98°
60	97°
50	96°

• ORAL ○ RECTAL

Respirations																									
Blood Pressure																									
Weight																									

	0700-1500	1500-2300	2300-0700	Total	0700-1500	1500-2300	2300-0700	Total	0700-1500	1500-2300	2300-0700	Total	0700-1500	1500-2300	2300-0700	Total	0700-1500	1500-2300	2300-0700	Total
Intake Oral																				
Parenteral																				
Total																				
Output Urine																				
Drainage																				
Emesis																				
Total																				
Stools																				

Figure 24-6

Reading a Kardex

The Kardex is a card file used in health care that contains information taken from the record or chart for daily care. It is a summary of the nursing plan and doctor's orders. The Kardex is a quick and easy reference and is completed in pencil so that the information may be updated as needed. Figure 24-7, A and B, represents a sample Kardex for a hospitalized patient. In the space provided, organize the tasks to be completed during the day shift.

Applying Your Knowledge

1. Explain whether it would be more efficient to organize the tasks by the type of task for more than one patient?

_____

_____

_____

2. What is the diagnosis for this patient?

_____

_____

_____

3. Why would it be acceptable or not be acceptable for this patient to walk to a day room and buy a snack?

_____

_____

_____

MODE OF ADMISSION: ED ☐ DIRECT ADMIT ☒ TRANSFER ☐

DATE	VITAL SIGN FREQUENCY	DATE	PERSONAL - ORAL HYGIENE	DATE	TREATMENTS	DATE	SPECIAL INSTRUCTIONS
5/30	T.P.R.: QID		COMPLETE:	5/30	Clinitest & Acetest q2hr ac & hs		
5/30	B.P.: QID		SELF WITH HELP:				
	NEURO CHECKS:		SELF CARE:				
			PERICARE:				
5/30	DAILY WT.:						
5/30	DIET: ADA 1800 Cal.		REHABILITATION SERVICES:				
	FLUID RESTRICTIONS:						
	TUBE FEEDING:						
							TEACHING:
	NG TUBE:		ACTIVITY:				
	SUCTION:		BED REST:				
	IRRIGATE:		BSC:				
			REPOSITION:				
	DRAINS/TUBES:		CHAIR:				
		5/30	UP AD LIB:				
			AMB. c̄ ASSIST				
5/30	INTAKE & OUTPUT:	5/30	SIDERAILS: ☐ FULL ☒ HALF		CENTRAL LINE CARE:		BOWEL/COLOSTOMY CARE:
	ROUTINE:		RELEASE SIGNED:				
	STRICT:			6/1	IV SITE (L)wrist CHANGE:		
	CATHETER: (TYPE)		RESTRAINTS:		IV SITE: CHANGE:		
	DC ___ ✓ VOIDING		☐ WRIST ☐ VEST		IV SITE: CHANGE:		
	IRRIGATION:		☐ 4 PT. LEATHERS				

Figure 24-7A

MODE OF TRANSPORT: AMBULATORY ☒ WHEELCHAIR ☐ CART ☐ BEDSIDE ☐   **MONITOR:** ☐ YES ☐ NO

DATE ORD'	DATE DONE	RESPIRATORY THERAPY	DATE ORD'	DATE DONE	MISCELLANEOUS	DATE ORD'	DATE DONE	LAB STUDIES	DATE ORD	DAILY STUDIES
		O² ___ LPM			ABG'S	5/30		ADMISSION: CBC	5/30	FBS
		MASK ___ T-PIECE ___ % O²						CPK/LDH		
		VENTILATOR FiO²						CHEM PROF I		
		TV ___ RATE						CPK - ISO Q12 HR X 3		
		MODE ___ PEEP						6 6 6		
		E.T. TUBE SIZE:								
		☐ NASAL ☐ ORAL								
		POSITION: cm								
		REPOSITIONED: cm								
		CHANGE/REINSERT								
		SPONTANEOUS PARAMETERS								
		RESP. TX:								SPECIMEN COLLECTION:
					EKG STUDIES:	5/30			5/30	UA ON ADMISSION
		X-RAY STUDIES			ADMISSION					
5/30		CXR ADMISSION			Q DAY 3					
		Q DAY X 3								
								BLOOD ON HOLD		
								ORD. ___ EXP. ___		

DATE ORD'	DATE DONE	SURGICAL & SPECIAL PROCEDURES		DATE NOT.	CONSULT/REFERRAL	SPEC.
6/2		Surgical fixation ℞ humerus		5/30	Diabetic teaching	
		PACER: LOCATION	REINSERT:			
		CVP: LOCATION	REINSERT:		SOCIAL SERVICE	
		A-LINE: LOCATION	REINSERT:		NUTRITIONAL SERVICES	
		SWAN: LOCATION			PATIENT EDUCATION	

ROOM	NAME	AGE	SEX	ADMITTING PHYSICIAN	ADMITTING DIAGNOSIS	RELIGION	ADM.DATE
402	Jayne, Beverly	45	F	Dolster, Wm.	Fx ℞ humerus		5/30

Figure 24-7B

271

Charting Practice

Review the guidelines for charting health care records found in Chapter 2 of the textbook. Figure 24-8 is a sample of charting written by a nurse assistant. In the space provided, list 10 of the guidelines for charting that were not followed. Rewrite the information provided in correct form in the space provided.

PATIENT PROGRESS NOTES

DATE	TIME	
5/30	2:30	Mrs. Jayne is an old battleax! She's refusing to eat her meals and complained all day. Her vital signs were okay at 8:15 and 1:30. She has ~~tmrte~~ trouble walking unless she's given help because she's so fat. There's some ~~bleeding~~ blood on the dressing on her ℞ arm —Susie Smith
		TEN GUIDELINES NOT FOLLOWED
	1.	
	2.	
	3.	
	4.	
	5.	
	6.	
	7.	
	8.	
	9.	
	10.	
		CORRECTED VERSION OF CHARTING

*SEE PATIENT PROGRESS NOTES FOR DESCRIPTION.   N/A APPLIES TO NOT APPLICABLE.

Figure 24-8

The following situations provide information for you to record. Chart the necessary information in the space provided in Figure 24-9, A and B. Use the charting guidelines found in Chapter 2 of the textbook as a reference for the correct method of charting.

PATIENT PROGRESS NOTES

DATE	TIME	

*SEE PATIENT PROGRESS NOTES FOR DESCRIPTION.   N/A APPLIES TO NOT APPLICABLE.

Figure 24-9A

PATIENT PROGRESS NOTES

DATE	TIME	

*SEE PATIENT PROGRESS NOTES FOR DESCRIPTION.   N/A APPLIES TO NOT APPLICABLE.

Figure 24-9B

Situation One

You have been providing care for Mrs. Jameson in room 434, bed 2. Mrs. Jameson is 65 years of age and has been in the hospital for surgery to replace the right hip joint. As you were instructed, you assisted her to walk to the end of the hall four times during your shift. She complained of feeling pain in the hip during the walks and placed a great deal of weight on you during the walks. During the day you assisted Mrs. Jameson to use the bedpan three times. Each time she was able to urinate only a small amount of cloudy, foul-smelling urine. She drank a cup of coffee and three glasses of juice during your shift. You also helped Mrs. Jameson take a shower using a shower chair. Mrs. Jameson talked to you several times during the day about her concern about taking care of herself at home when she is discharged because she lives alone.

Situation Two

You have provided care for Mr. Kennely during your shift. Mr. Kennely is 94 years of age and has pneumonia. He was admitted to the hospital in a confused state of mind. Mr. Kennely does not feed himself, so you assisted him to eat breakfast and lunch. He ate about half of both meals. You noticed that Mr. Kennely frequently has a productive cough. The sputum produced is yellowish gray. Mr. Kennely left his room and walked to the nurses' lounge during the shift. Once you had discovered that he had left the room, you looked for 5 minutes before finding him there. During the shift you assisted Mr. Kennely with a urinal several times. Mr. Kennely stated repeatedly that he needed to go out and work in his garden. He called you names and swore at you during all of the contacts you had with him.

Applying Your Knowledge

1. In both of the situations, describe any other action you would take in addition to charting your observations.

   _____

   _____

   _____

2. How might you improve the quality of care in each of the patient situations described?

   _____

   _____

   _____

Careers in Nursing

Nursing Skills and Qualities

List three personal qualities and skills that are important in nursing careers.

1. _____

2. _____

3. _____

Identifying Nursing Careers

Use the textbook to provide the missing information about nursing careers in Table 24-1.

TABLE 24-1 Nursing Careers

CAREER TITLE	YEARS OF EDUCATION	DESCRIPTION OF JOB DUTIES	CREDENTIALS REQUIRED
		Advanced practice, physical examinations, may prescribe medication, may practice independently	
			LPN, requires licensure to practice
		Supervise care of patients, work in a variety of settings	
	75 hours or more of training		
		Advanced nursing assistant skills in the patient's home	

Applying Your Knowledge

1. Confusion may occur with the background of this professional, who might complete a 2-, 3-, or 4-year degree to obtain the same license. This would describe the education of the _____.

2. The nurse who may deliver babies is called a _____.

3. An expanded role for the nurse assistant in the community may describe the

   _____.

4. The registered nurse who completes additional training and education may be called a

   _____.

5. The health care worker who works under the supervision of a registered nurse or licensed practical nurse to give daily care is called the _____.

Understanding Vital Signs

Figure 24-10 is an example of a graphic sheet of vital signs completed for Mrs. Martha Jewel during a 5-day hospital stay.

GRAPHIC RECORD
SIDE A

Jewel, Martha
Nelson, Douglas, M.D.
Room 506
Appendicitis

DATE	1-15-10						1-16-10						1-17-10						1-18-10						1-19-10					
HOSPITAL DAYS	-Admit-						-2-						-3-						-4-						-5-					
P.O. DAY	–						–						-1-						-2-											
	AM			PM			AM			PM			AM			PM			AM			PM			AM			PM		
HOUR	4	8	12	4	8	12	4	8	12	4	8	12	4	8	12	4	8	12	4	8	12	4	8	12	4	8	12	4	8	12

(Temperature graph: To Surgery; Discharged)

PULSE				88	84	76																								
RESPIRATION				20	18	16																								
BLOOD PRESSURE				134/84	130/80	124/74																								

HEIGHT	WT. 125 lb.	WT.	WT.	WT.	WT.
24 HR. TOTAL INTAKE	500 cc+	Parenteral-900 cc 100 cc+	850 cc	650 cc	
24 HR. TOTAL OUTPUT	700 cc+	850 cc	780 cc	700 cc	
STOOL				Formed, Brown	
STOOL FOR GUAIAC	—	—	—	—	—

Figure 24-10

Examining the Evidence

1. Why was Mrs. Jewel admitted to the hospital?

_____

_____

_____

2. When did Mrs. Jewel run a fever during her stay?

_____

_____

_____

3. When was the highest blood pressure reading taken during Mrs. Jewel's stay?

_____

_____

_____

4. On which postoperative day did Mrs. Jewel leave the hospital?

_____

_____

_____

5. When were the vital signs for Mrs. Jewel omitted during her stay?

_____

_____

_____

6. What is the name of Mrs. Jewel's doctor?

_____

_____

_____

Education and Career Research

Use the following links, other Internet resources, and information available by telephone or mail inquiry to determine the educational cost of one nursing career and the salary that might be earned in the local area. Use the information to complete Table 24-2.

Suggested Websites

Salary.com: http://salary.com
Monster.com: http://monster.com
Occupational Outlook Handbook: http://www.bls.gov/oco/
American Nurses Association: http://www.nursingworld.org/

TABLE 24-2 Education and Career Research

CAREER	INSTITUTION FOR EDUCATION	COST OF EDUCATION	POTENTIAL EARNINGS

Funeral Preparation

Use the Internet to explore the cost and options of funeral arrangements that reflect your cultural and religious beliefs. Write an essay that explains your thoughts about death and treatment of the body following death.

Essay

_____

_____

_____

_____

_____

_____

_____

_____

_____

_____

_____

_____

_____

_____

_____

_____

_____

_____

_____

_____

_____

_____

_____

_____

_____

_____

_____

_____

_____

_____

_____

_____

_____

_____

25 Medical Careers

VAPID VOCABULARY

Complete the crossword puzzle using the Key Terms.

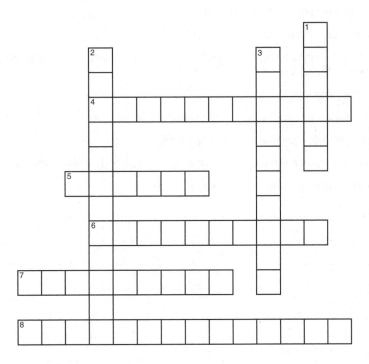

ACROSS

4 Treatment of disease and injury with an emphasis on the relationship between the body organs and musculoskeletal system
5 Clearness or sharpness of perception
6 Treatment of disease and injury with active intervention
7 Period of training in a specific area under the supervision of a qualified health care practitioner
8 Study of medicine to relieve pain during surgery

DOWN

1 Capacity for sight
2 Study of the mechanical laws and their application to living organisms, especially locomotion
3 Period of initial training under the supervision of a qualified practitioner

Match each of the following abbreviations with the phrase that best describes its meaning or function. Then write the phrase or name for each of the abbreviations in the spaces provided.

Abbreviation	**Meaning or Function**
1. _____ ABMS	a. Health care worker who often helps a doctor in the office
2. _____ CMA	b. Health care worker who helps a doctor in the office and is certified
3. _____ CST	c. Health care worker who assists surgeons
4. _____ DO	d. Health care worker who examines and tests eyes
5. _____ ECG	e. Health care worker who extends a doctor's ability to care for patients in the hospital, office, or surgery
6. _____ MA	
7. _____ MD	f. Operating room assistant who is certified
8. _____ OD	g. Organization that certifies doctors in specialties
9. _____ PA	h. Physicians who emphasize treatment of disease
10. _____ ST	i. Physicians who emphasize treatment of the overall body and movement
	j. Test that shows the electrical activity of the heart

1. ABMS: _____

2. CMA: _____

3. CST: _____

4. DO: _____

5. ECG: _____

6. MA: _____

7. MD: _____

8. OD: _____

9. PA: _____

10. ST: _____

1. There are two types of medical doctors, the MD (Doctor of _ _ _ _ _ _ _ _) and the DO (Doctor of Ⓞ _ _ _ _ _ _ _ _ _ _ _ Medicine).

2. Additional training under the supervision of a practicing doctor is needed for medical school graduates to specialize and includes an _ _ _ _ _ _ _ _ _ _ _ or _ _ _ _ _ _ _ _ _ _ _.

3. _ _ _ _ _ _ _ _ _ _ _ _ _ _ _ _ _ _ are medical doctors who diagnose and treat diseases and injuries of the eyes.

4. The role of the _ _ _ _ _ Ⓞ _ _ _ assistant was developed to relieve some of the tasks performed by the medical doctor to extend the availability of care.

5. Ⓞ _ _ _ _ _ _ _ _ _ _ are eye muscle specialists who work under the direction of an ophthalmologist.

6. _ _ _ _ _ _ _ Ⓞ technologists assist during surgical operations under the supervision of the surgeon and registered nurse.

7. The _ _ _ _ _ _ _ assistant performs both clerical and clinical functions under the supervision of a physician.

8. _ _ _ _ _ _ _ _ _ _ _ _ is the ability to differentiate shapes and colors to interpret their meaning.

9. The medical or optometric assistant, using a _ _ _ _ _ _ _ _ _ _ Ⓞ _ that measures the ability to see symbols from a specified distance, may test vision.

10. While assisting with the physical examination, the medical assistant may take
_ _ _ _ _ _ _ _ _ _ and _ _ _ _ _ the patient.

Use the circled letters to form the answer to this jumble. Clue: What about a package indicates that it has been sterilized?

_ _ _ _ _

Reviewing Structures of Anatomy

Use Chapters 10 through 21 to identify each of the structures of the body in Figure 25-1, A to E. List the body system and function of each structure in Table 25-1.

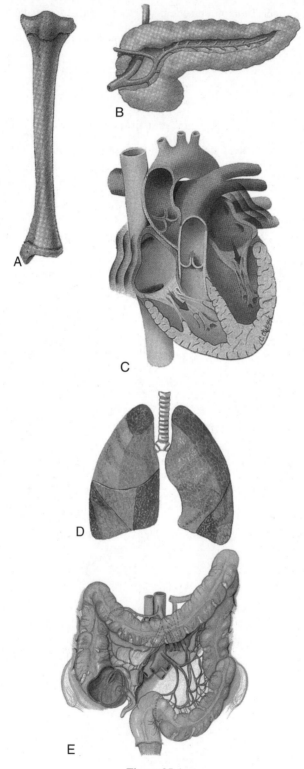

Figure 25-1

TABLE 25-1 Anatomy Structures

BODY STRUCTURE	SYSTEM	FUNCTION
A.		
B.		
C.		
D.		
E.		

Medical Careers

Medical Skills and Qualities

List three personal qualities and skills that are important in medical careers.

1. _____

2. _____

3. _____

Identifying Medical Careers

Use the textbook to provide the missing information about medical careers in Table 25-2.

TABLE 25-2 Medical Careers

CAREER TITLE	YEARS OF EDUCATION	DESCRIPTION OF JOB DUTIES AND OPPORTUNITIES	CREDENTIALS REQUIRED
		Use corrective devices, surgery, and medication to treat disorders of the foot	
			OD, licensed by the state
		Anesthesiology, urology, obstetrics, surgery, pediatrics, and other specialties; private practice or employment by hospital or clinic	
			DC, licensed by the state
		Work under the supervision of a physician to perform similar duties	

Applying Your Knowledge

1. The health care workers who are eye muscle specialists and who complete 24 months of training following 2 years of college are called _____.

2. A technique that originated with the Chinese and is now performed by health practitioners is called

   _____.

3. The health practitioner who helps the physician and trains for 1 to 2 years is called the

   _____.

4. Medical doctors who treat disorders of the eyes are called _____.

5. Following licensure or certification by the state, one of the health care practitioners who also must complete at least 100 hours of continuing education every 6 years is called the _____.

INVESTIGATIONS

Sterilizing Packages

Read all of the directions before beginning this activity. Sterilization is the process used to kill all microorganisms on an object. Laboratory activities should be completed under the supervision of a qualified professional only.

Equipment and Supplies

Autoclave
Autoclave tape
Autoclave paper or lint-free towel
Metal instrument for sterilization

Directions

1. Maintain medical asepsis by using good handwashing technique. Wrapping packages for sterilization is a clean procedure that requires the hands and instruments to be as free of microorganisms as possible.
2. Select clean instruments for sterilization. Instruments may be arranged into sets for convenient use in particular procedures.
3. Select a wrapping towel or drape that is large enough to cover all contents completely. Drapes for autoclave sterilization may be made of cotton or specialized disposable material. Draping materials must allow penetration by the pressurized steam or gas.
4. Place instrumentation and sterilizing indicator diagonally in the center of the wrapping material. The outside indicating tape does not ensure that the inner contents have been sterilized.
5. Fold the corners of the draping material into the center of the tray. The near edge is folded first, sides next, and the far side last. The package should be neat and tight with no exposed edges of the wrapping material. Tuck the last edge into the pocket formed by the first three sides.
6. Seal the package with indicator tape. Secure the tape so that the package will not be pulled open when the tape is removed.
7. Label the tape with the date and time of sterilization, contents, and the initials of the preparer. Items are not considered sterile indefinitely and must be resterilized if not used within a reasonable length of time.
8. Place the package in the appropriate location for articles needing sterilization or load it into the autoclave.
9. Load clean glassware, instruments, or packages into the autoclave with containers and clasps open. Insert the indicator tape or pellet. Supplies may be wrapped in muslin, paper, nylon, or cellophane or in a sealing package before sterilization. During autoclaving, closed containers may explode as a result of the expansion of trapped air. Clasps must be opened to allow sterilization of all surface areas. Wrappers must be made of material that allows penetration by the steam heat.
10. Close and latch the autoclave door.
11. Steam the items for 20 minutes at 20 pounds of pressure at 275° F. The necessary time for sterilization may differ, depending on the size of the load in the autoclave.
12. Allow the pressure of the autoclave to return to zero before opening the door. The pressure reading must be at zero before opening the autoclave to avoid rapid release of steam and possible injury.
13. Remove the sterile equipment or packages and store them in the appropriate location. Individually sterilized articles must be removed with another sterile instrument to prevent contamination.

286

Drawing Conclusions

1. Why is it important to place a sterilization indicator inside the package as well as outside?

   _____

   _____

   _____

2. Ethylene oxide gas is used to sterilize materials such as plastics and rubber. Why is steam sterilization not used for these materials?

   _____

   _____

   _____

CRITICAL THINKING

Medical Detecting

This activity is adapted from the VQI (Vector Quest 1) series developed by the Iowa Medical Foundation. It allows you to be an epidemiologist or medical detective. Use the case study to answer the questions.

The Last Case

Janet Parker was very British. She loved tennis at Wimbledon, tea in the afternoon, the white cliffs of Dover, and Monty Python's Flying Circus. In 1978, Ms. Parker died a very un-British death. After becoming severely ill with a high fever and a rash, Ms. Parker died within 5 days. She died from what doctors said could only have been smallpox. Her death occurred 5 years after Britain had reported its last case of this disease.

Ms. Parker had been a medical photographer employed at the University of Birmingham. One week after Ms. Parker's death, her mother was diagnosed as having the last case of smallpox in Britain. Her mother survived. Neither Janet nor her mother had ever traveled to Africa, where earlier that year the world's last case was prematurely documented.

Regrettably, 1 week after Janet Parker's death, Professor Henry Bedson of the University of Birmingham committed suicide. Professor Bedson had been the head of the University's Microbiology and Virology Department.

In 1978 the World Health Organization, with help from more than 200,000 health officers and volunteers, won one of mankind's greatest battles. Smallpox was the first disease to be eradicated by human effort. Ironically, Janet Parker, one of its last victims, was from a country that had eradicated the disease years earlier.

Examining the Evidence

1. What questions would you like answered to help determine the source of Janet Parker's illness?

   _____

   _____

   _____

2. Describe the variables that might be involved in Janet Parker's illness.

   _____

   _____

   _____

3. What could have been the vector for Janet Parker's illness?

_____

_____

_____

4. What are four things that can be done by every person to prevent the spread of disease?

_____

_____

_____

5. In your opinion, would it be better to keep or destroy any remaining samples of smallpox that exist?

_____

_____

_____

The Case of the Red Rings

In the summer of 1988, Jeffrey Donner of Waysata, Minnesota, was having a typical vacation filled with swimming, cycling, a camping trip with his Scout group, a family trip, and baseball. On July 14, Jeffrey came down with what his family thought was the flu. He had a fever, chills, swollen glands, fatigue, head and body aches, a sore throat, and nausea.

Within a 50-mile radius of his home, 78 other people were suffering from the same disease. Ten percent of these people went on to develop cardiac problems, and 15% experienced severe nerve problems.

In talking with Jeffrey, health care professionals discovered that prior to his symptoms, he had noticed a "ring-like rash" on his lower legs. This bright red mark was approximately 10 cm, or 4 inches, wide and was itchy and painful.

Approximately half of the nearly 80 cases of this disease developed arthritic-like conditions within 1 year of the early symptoms. This result was unusual because the victims ranged in age from 3 to 84 years.

Examining the Evidence

1. What questions would you like answered to help determine the source of Jeffrey's illness?

_____

_____

_____

2. Describe the variables that might be involved in Jeffrey's illness.

_____

_____

_____

3. What could have been the vector for Jeffrey's illness?

_____

_____

_____

4. How could the spread of this vector be stopped?

_____

_____

_____

INTERNET ACTIVITIES

Education and Career Research

Use the following links, other Internet resources, and information available by telephone or mail inquiry to determine the educational cost of one medical career and the salary that might be earned in the local area. Use the information to complete Table 25-3.

Suggested Websites

Salary.com: http://salary.com
Monster.com: http://monster.com
Occupational Outlook Handbook: http://www.bls.gov/oco/
American Medical Association: http://www.ama-assn.org/ama/pub/education-careers/careers-health-care.shtml
The American Association of Medical Assistants: http://www.aama-ntl.org/

TABLE 25-3 Education and Career Research

CAREER	INSTITUTION FOR EDUCATION	COST OF EDUCATION	POTENTIAL EARNINGS

Chapter **25 Medical Careers**

VAPID VOCABULARY

Complete the crossword puzzle using the Key Terms.

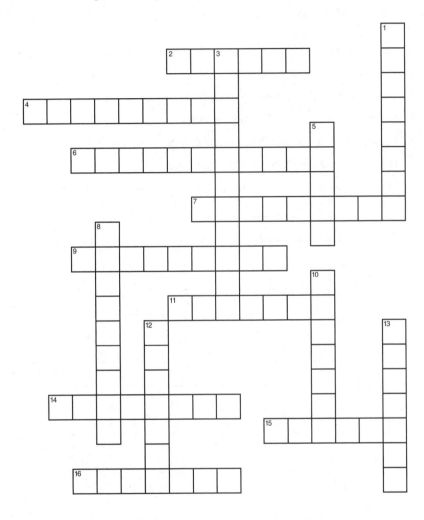

ACROSS

2 Decalcification of the surface of the tooth followed by disintegration of the inner part of the tooth; cavity
4 The teeth that erupt first and are replaced by permanent dentition; primary teeth
6 Situated or occurring around a tooth
7 Offensive or bad breath
9 Used to designate natural teeth in the mouth
11 Gum of the mouth, mucous membrane with supporting fibrous tissue
14 Bone of the lower jaw
15 Mass adhering to the enamel surface of a tooth, composed of mixed bacterial colonies and organic material
16 Bony cavities in maxilla and mandible in which the roots of the teeth are attached

DOWN

1 Calcium phosphate and carbonate with organic matter, deposited on the surfaces of teeth; tartar
3 Replacement of part of a tooth, usually with silver alloy, gold, or aesthetic composite material
5 Solid mixture of two or more metals
8 The teeth that erupt and take the place of deciduous dentition; secondary teeth
10 Irregularly shaped bone that forms the upper jaw
12 Proper care of the mouth and teeth for maintenance of health and the prevention of disease
13 Localized collection of pus in a cavity formed by destruction of tissue

ABBREVIATIONS

Match each of the following abbreviations with the phrase that best describes its meaning or function. Then write the phrase or name for each of the abbreviations in the spaces provided.

Abbreviation

1. _____ ADA
2. _____ CDL
3. _____ DA
4. _____ DDS
5. _____ DH
6. _____ DLT
7. _____ DMD
8. _____ NADL
9. _____ NCRP
10. _____ RDH

Meaning or Function

a. Certified dental worker who makes bridges and other prostheses

b. Dental worker who makes bridges and other prostheses

c. Dental worker who may answer the phone as well as help the dentist during examinations

d. Dental worker who may provide dental care independently or assist a dentist

e. Hygienist who earns advanced standing through registration

f. One of two doctoral degrees for dentists

g. One of two doctoral degrees for dentists

h. Organization that adopted the universal system of numbering teeth

i. Organization that certifies dental lab technicians

j. Organization that sets the standards for radiation exposure for dental workers

1. ADA: _____

2. CDL: _____

3. DA: _____

4. DDS: _____

5. DH: _____

6. DLT: _____

7. DMD: _____

8. NADL: _____

9. NCRP: _____

10. RDH: _____

1. The dental team includes the _ _ _ _ _ ◯ _, dental _ _ _ _ _ _ _ _ _ _, dental _ _ _ ◯ _ _ _ _ _ _, and dental _ _ _ _ _ _ _ _ _ _ technician.

2. Dentists perform a variety of services, including _ _ _ _ _ _ education, detection of ◯ _ _ _ _ _ _ _, _ _ _ _ _ _ _ _ improvement of appearance, and correction of ◯ _ _ _ problems.

3. Some of the _ _ _ _ _ specialties that dentists may practice include endodontics, orthodontics, and periodontics.

4. Some areas in which the dental _ _ _ _ _ _ _ _ ◯ may specialize include clinical work, education, administration, research, consumer advocacy, or veterinary dental practice.

5. The dental _ _ _ _ _ _ _ _ _' _ responsibilities may include answering the telephone, making appointments, and working with billing accounts.

6. Dental _ _ _ ◯ _ _ _ _ _ _ _ _ ◯ _ _ _ _ _ _ _ are the only members of the dental health care team who do not work directly with patients.

7. ◯ _ _ _ _ _ _ _ _ _ _ disease is caused by infection in the supporting structures of teeth, such as the gingiva and bones.

8. Functions of the teeth include the mechanical portion of _ _ _ _ _ _ _ _ _, _ _ _ _ _ of the face, and aiding the production of _ _ ◯ _ _ _.

9. The tooth is divided into two sections called the _ _ _ _ ◯ and _ _ _ _.

10. The descriptive anatomy of the tooth is called _ ◯ _ _ _ _ _ _ _ _.

Use the circled letters to form the answer to this jumble. Clue: What is the practice of dentistry that provides care for children?

_ _ _ _ _ _ _ _ _ _ _ _

Identifying Structures of the Oral Cavity

Use Figure 26-8 of the textbook to label the diagram of the oral cavity in Figure 26-1.

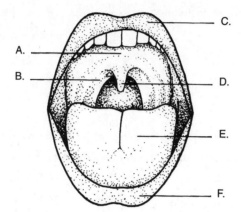

Figure 26-1

A. _____   D. _____

B. _____   E. _____

C. _____   F. _____

Identifying Structures of the Tooth

Use Figure 26-10 of the textbook to label the diagram of the tooth in Figure 26-2.

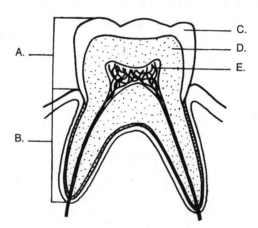

Figure 26-2

A. _____   D. _____

B. _____   E. _____

C. _____

Identifying the Teeth in the Mouth

Use Figure 26-9 of the textbook to label the diagrams of the teeth in the mouth in Figure 26-3.

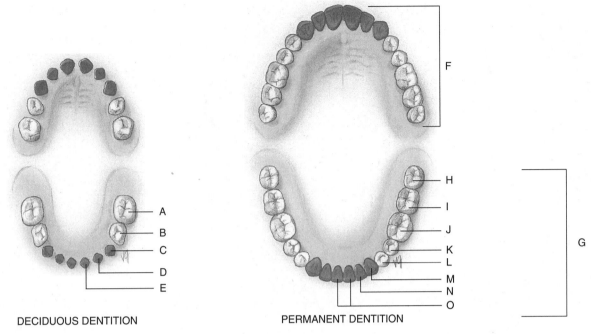

DECIDUOUS DENTITION

PERMANENT DENTITION

Figure 26-3

A. _____

B. _____

C. _____

D. _____

E. _____

F. _____

G. _____

H. _____

I. _____

J. _____

K. _____

L. _____

M. _____

N. _____

O. _____

Identifying Surfaces of the Teeth

Use Figure 26-11 of the textbook to label the diagram of the surfaces of a tooth in Figure 26-4.

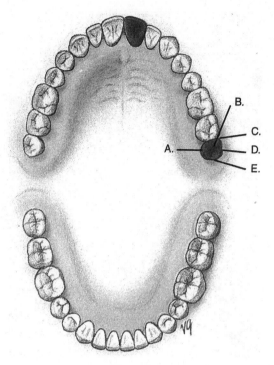

Figure 26-4

A. _____   D. _____

B. _____   E. _____

C. _____

Charting Dental Structures

Mrs. Smith, a 62-year-old woman, has the dental history shown in Table 26-1. Use Figure 26-12 of the textbook to chart the information regarding Mrs. Smith's dentition in Figure 26-5.

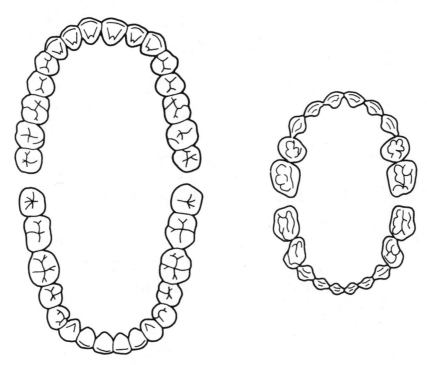

Figure 26-5

TOOTH NUMBER	DENTAL STRUCTURE
1	Tooth missing
2	Amalgam restoration
3	Amalgam restoration
14	Esthetic restoration
15	Gold crown
16	Tooth missing
17	Amalgam restoration
18	Caries or decay
31	Root canal
32	Gold crown

Drawing Conclusions

1. Why is it normal for the third molars to be missing?

_____

_____

_____

2. Why would Mrs. Smith need a dental visit?

_____

_____

_____

Dental Careers

Dental Skills and Qualities

List three personal qualities and skills that are important in dental careers.

1. _____

2. _____

3. _____

Identifying Dental Careers

Use the textbook to provide the missing information about dental careers in Table 26-1.

TABLE 26-1 Dental Careers

CAREER TITLE	YEARS OF EDUCATION	DESCRIPTION OF JOB DUTIES AND OPPORTUNITIES	CREDENTIALS REQUIRED
	No educational standards set, 1-2 years training		
			DDS or DMD, licensure required
		Scope of practice varies greatly; cleans teeth, records patient history, takes radiographs, teaches dental hygiene, administers anesthesia	
	On-the-job training or college program	Makes dental prostheses	

Applying Your Knowledge

1. The health care worker who applies braces to correct misalignment of teeth is called a _____.

2. The health care worker who gives instruction on how to floss teeth is the _____.

3. Dental radiographs may be taken by two different workers, including the _____

   and the _____.

4. The health care worker who cleans the teeth below the gum is the _____.

5. After an accident, surgery to correct injuries would probably be performed by the _____.

Practicing Oral Hygiene

Read all of the directions before beginning this activity. Laboratory activities should be completed under the supervision of a qualified professional only.

Equipment and Supplies

Dental floss
Disclosing tablet
Mirror
Toothbrush
Toothpaste

Directions

1. Practice medical asepsis by using good handwashing technique.
2. Brush your teeth for 3 minutes using a toothbrush and toothpaste of preference.
3. Floss your teeth as instructed in the textbook.
4. Chew a disclosing tablet provided by your instructor.
5. Use a mirror to identify the areas missed during brushing and flossing.
6. Brush your teeth to remove all color remaining from the tablet.

Drawing Conclusions

1. Which areas of your teeth, if any, did you omit in brushing?

   _____

   _____

   _____

2. Why would it be more likely for a cavity to form on a tooth that is habitually missed during brushing?

   _____

   _____

   _____

Practicing Dental Identification

Read all of the directions before beginning this activity. Laboratory activities should be completed under the supervision of a qualified professional only.

Equipment and Supplies

Dental floss
Toothbrush
Toothpaste

Directions

1. Practice medical asepsis by using good handwashing technique.
2. Brush and floss your teeth using the instructions in the textbook.
3. With a partner, use the instructions in the textbook to chart each student's dental history in Figure 26-6.
4. Hold your mouth open wide for another student to see and chart the dental structures and restorations visible. You may use your fingers to hold your mouth open wide. *Note:* Each student should place only his or her own fingers in the mouth.

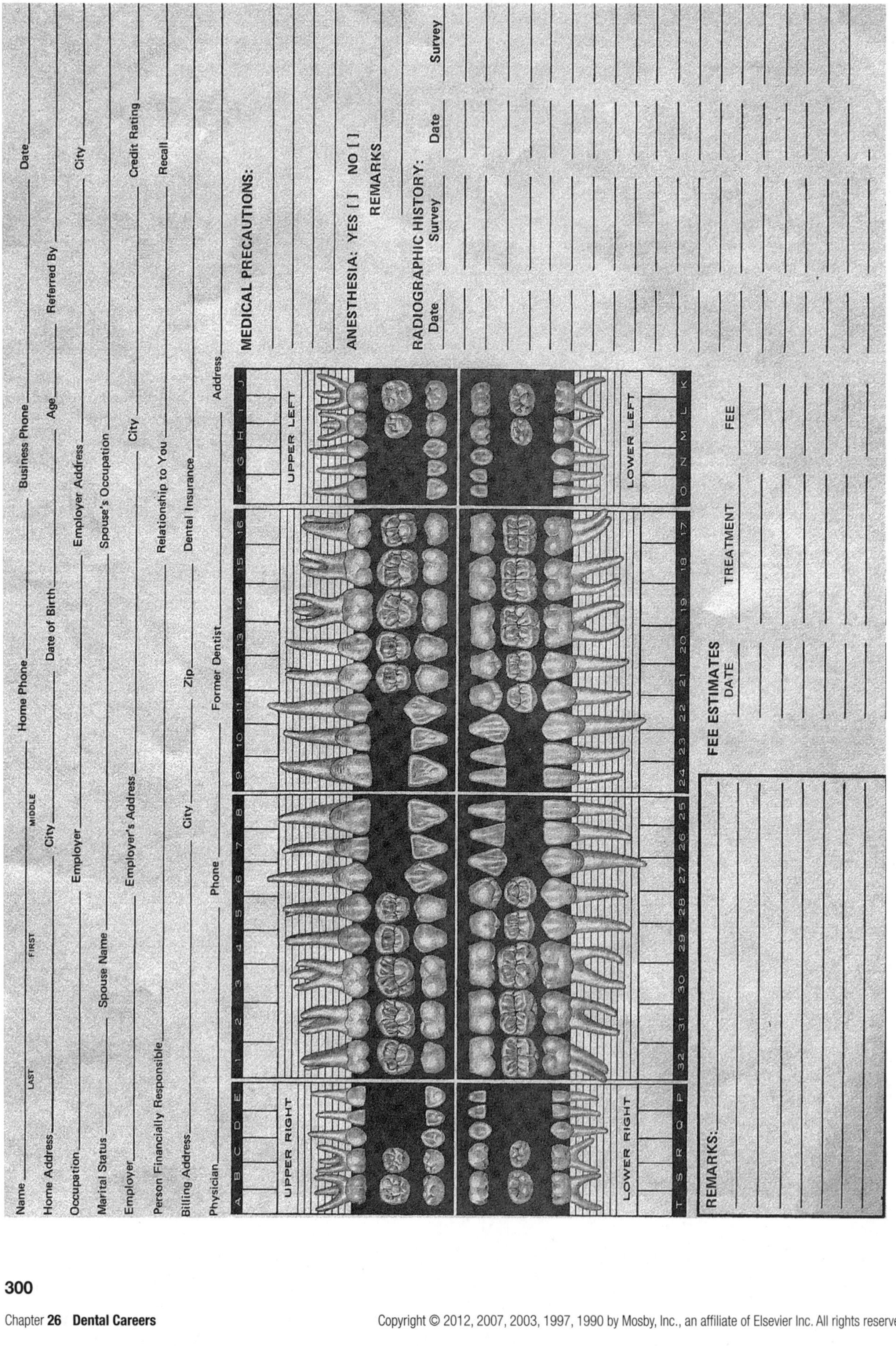

Name ___ LAST ___ FIRST ___ MIDDLE ___ Date ___

Home Phone ___ Business Phone ___

Home Address ___ City ___

Date of Birth ___ Age ___ Referred By ___

Occupation ___ Employer ___ Employer Address ___ City ___

Marital Status ___ Spouse Name ___ Spouse's Occupation ___

Employer ___ Employer's Address ___ City ___ Credit Rating ___

Person Financially Responsible ___ Relationship to You ___ Recall ___

Billing Address ___ City ___ Zip ___ Dental Insurance ___

Physician ___ Phone ___ Former Dentist ___ Address ___

MEDICAL PRECAUTIONS:

ANESTHESIA: YES [ ] NO [ ] REMARKS ___

RADIOGRAPHIC HISTORY:

Date ___ Survey ___ Date ___ Survey ___ Date ___ Survey ___

UPPER RIGHT   UPPER LEFT

A B C D E 1 2 3 4 5 6 7 8 9 10 11 12 13 14 15 16 F G H I J

LOWER RIGHT   LOWER LEFT

T S R Q P 32 31 30 29 28 27 26 25 24 23 22 21 20 19 18 17 O N M L K

FEE ESTIMATES

DATE	TREATMENT	FEE

REMARKS:

Figure 26-6A

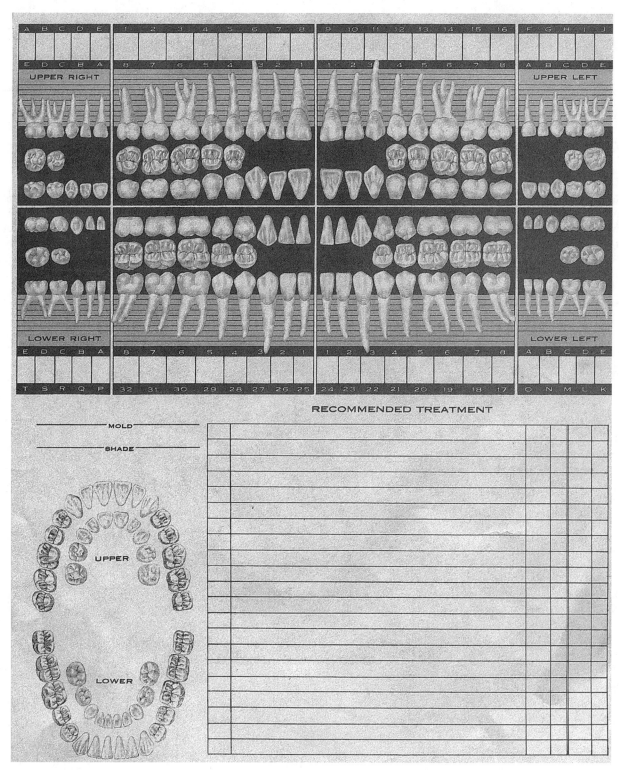

Figure 26-6B

Drawing Conclusions

1. Why should each student place only his or her own fingers in the mouth?

_____

_____

_____

CRITICAL THINKING

Dental Phobia

More than an estimated 40 million Americans suffer from some degree of dental phobia, or an irrational fear of dental examination. Symptoms of this problem include anxiety and physiological changes related to stress. Some techniques have been developed to reduce the phobia related to dental appointments, including resisting the negative thoughts about the visit before seeing the dentist. It has also been demonstrated that it may be helpful for the patient to focus on taking regular breaths during the visit and to inform the dentist when fear is present. Focusing on positive thoughts, such as "I am getting good care and improving my health," also may be helpful.

Examining the Evidence

1. Why do you think some people experience dental phobia?

_____

_____

_____

2. What other suggestions could you make to reduce the anxiety of the dental visit?

_____

_____

_____

3. What could a health care worker do in the office to reduce the dental phobia of the patient?

_____

_____

_____

4. What other statements could be used to generate positive thoughts and promote concentration during the appointment?

_____

_____

_____

5. Why is it important to communicate the fear of a dental visit to the dentist?

_____

_____

_____

Is Gum Good?

Some types of chewing gum actually help prevent tooth decay. Xylitol, a sweetener made from cornstalks, helps seal caries. A 3-year study to test the role of xylitol in tooth decay, which involved 1200 children between the ages of 9 and 11 years, was conducted by Kauko K. Makinen, a biochemist at the University of Michigan, who reached this conclusion. The experiment involved having the children chew gum three to five times a day for several minutes. Some gums used contained xylitol, whereas others contained sucrose (sugar) or sorbitol (another artificial sweetener).

The study showed a slightly higher increase in tooth decay in children who chewed gum with sucrose than in those who did not chew gum at all. Both of these gums showed a greater increase in the number of caries than was seen in the children who chewed gum with sorbitol. However, a comparable decrease was found in the number of caries in children who chewed gum with xylitol.

Makinen also reported that bacteria that cause caries do not break down xylitol into acids. Because the xylitol is not broken down into acids, the bacteria do not cause decay.

Examining the Evidence

1. What controls did Makinen use in the study concerning gum sweeteners?

   _____

   _____

   _____

2. How could this study be duplicated?

   _____

   _____

   _____

3. Visualize and describe an advertisement for print or audio to sell a gum containing xylitol.

   _____

   _____

   _____

4. In more than one mystery story, the culprit is caught by matching the indentations of his or her teeth that were found at the scene of the crime, in foods such as cheese or even gum. Is this a realistic scenario?

   _____

   _____

   _____

Education and Career Research

Use the following links, other Internet resources, and information available by telephone or mail inquiry to determine the educational cost of one dental career and the salary that might be earned in the local area. Use the information to complete Table 26-2.

Suggested Websites

Salary.com: http://salary.com
Monster.com: http://monster.com
Occupational Outlook Handbook: http://www.bls.gov/oco/
American Dental Association: http://www.ada.org/
American Dental Hygienists' Association: http://www.adha.org/
American Dental Assistant Association: http://www.dentalassistant.org/

TABLE 26-2 Education and Career Research

CAREER	INSTITUTION FOR EDUCATION	COST OF EDUCATION	POTENTIAL EARNINGS

Complementary and Alternative Careers

VAPID VOCABULARY

Complete the crossword puzzle using the Key Terms.

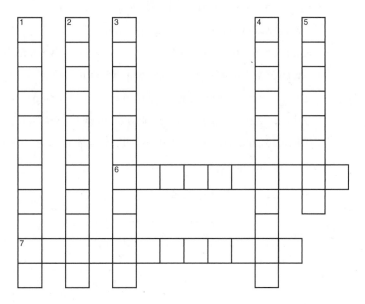

ACROSS

6 System of medical practice that uses remedies designed to produce effects that are different than those caused by the disease being treated

7 System of therapy based on the theory that health is determined by the condition of the nervous system

DOWN

1 Conscious control of biological functions normally controlled involuntarily

2 System of medical practice that uses remedies designed to produce similar effects to those caused by the disease being treated

3 Incomplete dislocation of a joint

4 Dose of a vitamin

5 Practice of medicine that considers the person as a whole unit, not as individual parts

ABBREVIATIONS

Match each of the following abbreviations with the phrase that best describes its meaning or function. Then write the phrase or name for each of the abbreviations in the spaces provided.

Abbreviation	Meaning or Function
1. _____ AANP	a. Doctors who treat problems associated with the musculoskeletal and nervous systems
2. _____ ACA	b. Organization that approves schools of massage
3. _____ AMTA	c. Organization that certifies biofeedback practitioners
4. _____ BCIA	d. Organization that certifies chiropractors
5. _____ CAM	e. Organization that divides CAM treatments into five domains
6. _____ CHT	f. Organization that is the professional group for naturopathic doctors
7. _____ DC	g. Organization that provides grants to test CAM treatments
8. _____ NCCAM	h. Primary care physicians who focus on the whole person
9. _____ ND	i. Therapies and treatments that go with or instead of traditional medical care
10. _____ NIH	j. Type of alternative treatment

1. AANP: _____

2. ACA: _____

3. AMTA: _____

4. BCIA: _____

5. CAM: _____

6. CHT: _____

7. DC: _____

8. NCCAM: _____

9. ND: _____

10. NIH: _____

JUST THE FACTS

1. Complementary medicine is a therapy based on __ __ __ __ __ __ __ __ and __ __ ⬤ __ __ __ __
   treatment.

2. Based on a 2007 survey, the NIH reported that more than 38% of Americans use therapies outside of
   __ __ __ __ __ __ ⬤ __ __ __ medicine.

3. The National Institutes of Health groups CAM practices into __ __ ⬤ __ __ __ __ __ __ __ __ __.

4. __ __ __ __ __ __ __ __ __ __ __ ⬤ __ __ __ treat health problems associated with the muscular,
   skeletal, and nervous systems.

5. ◯_ _ _ _ _ _ _ _ _ _ _ _ _ doctors are primary care physicians who focus on the treatment of the whole person, with emphasis on wellness and disease prevention.

6. _ _ _ _ _ ◯ _　_ _ _ _ _ _ _ ◯ _ _ _ use skillful touch to loosen muscles and relieve pain.

7. _ _ _ _ _ _ _ _ _ _ _ _ _ _ _ _ insert needles into peripheral or surface nerves to control pain, provide anesthesia, relieve symptoms, and modify psychosomatic disorders.

8. _ ◯ _ _ _ _ _ _ _ _ _ is a technique used to change normally involuntary reactions of the body using conscious control.

9. _ _ _ _ _ _ ◯ _ _ _ _ medicine is a Western system based on the concept that "like cures like."

10. Many of the biologically based therapies considered to be CAM overlap with conventional medicine and involve special _ _ ◯ _ _ _ _ _　_ _ _ _ _ _ _ _ ◯ _ _ _ or programs.

   Use the circled letters to form the answer to this jumble. Clue: What are the nonallopathic practices that have been proven to be effective by research called?

_ _ _ _ _ _ _ _ _ _ _ _ _

CONCEPT APPLICATIONS

Describing the Domains of CAM
Describe each of the five categories or domains of complementary and alternative medicine.

1. Whole medical systems

   _____

   _____

   _____

2. Manipulative and body-based methods

   _____

   _____

   _____

3. Mind-body interventions

   _____

   _____

   _____

4. Biologically based therapy

   _____

   _____

   _____

5. Energy therapy

_____

_____

_____

Complementary and Alternative Careers

Complementary and Alternative Skills and Qualities

List three personal qualities and skills that are important in complementary and alternative careers.

1. _____

2. _____

3. _____

Identifying Complementary and Alternative Careers

Use the textbook to provide the missing information about complementary and alternative careers in Table 27-1.

TABLE 27-1 Complementary and Alternative Careers

CAREER TITLE	YEARS OF EDUCATION	DESCRIPTION OF JOB DUTIES AND OPPORTUNITIES	CREDENTIALS REQUIRED
	Minimum of 2 years of college and completion of a 4- to 5-year program		
		Insertion of needles into peripheral nerves to control pain, provide alternative, and relieve symptoms	
Naturopathic doctor			
			Licensure required in 13 states
			Certification available for applicants licensed or working under the supervision of a licensed health care practitioner

Applying Your Knowledge

1. The practitioner who adjusts the spine to correct disorders is the _____.

2. A practitioner who helps the patient overcome bad habits and treats emotional problems is the

   _____.

3. The CAM practitioner who holds a medical degree but does not prescribe medications is the _____

   _____.

4. The CAM practitioner who uses a technique believed to release endorphins into the blood stream is the

   _____.

5. Manipulation of the skin, muscles, tendons, and ligaments is a therapeutic technique of the _____

   _____.

INVESTIGATIONS

Using Biofeedback to Measure and Control Body Reactions

Read all of the instructions before beginning this activity. Laboratory activities should be completed under the supervision of a qualified professional only.

Equipment and Supplies

Liquid crystal thermal indicator (Biodot)

Directions

1. Wash and dry both hands thoroughly.
2. Apply a liquid crystal thermal indicator to the flap between the thumb and index finger on the hand that is not dominant.
3. Note the color of the Biodot in Table 27-2.
4. Monitor the color of the Biodot throughout the rest of the day, noting the time and activity of any color change. Data collection is complete when the Biodot becomes dislodged.
5. Record the information in Table 27-2 for any color change that occurs.

TABLE 27-2 Biofeedback Reactions

TIME OF READING	COLOR OF BIODOT	ACTIVITY
Initial =		

Drawing Conclusions

1. What type of activity was the most stressful, using the Biodot as the indicator of your stress level?

   _____

   _____

   _____

Chapter **27** **Complementary and Alternative Careers**

2. Did you feel most stressed during the activity indicated to be stressful by the Biodot?

_____

_____

_____

3. What are some other factors that might influence the reading of the Biodot?

_____

_____

_____

4. What are some other measurements that could indicate increased stress that would be more reliable than the Biodot?

_____

_____

_____

5. What type of relaxation technique could you use during stressful activities?

_____

_____

_____

CRITICAL THINKING

Understanding Clinical Trials

Using the following Internet link, read about clinical trials in CAM being conducted by the National Institutes of Health. Then answer the following questions.

http://nccam.nih.gov/research/clinicaltrials/

1. What is a clinical trial?

_____

_____

_____

2. What are the common elements of a clinical trial?

_____

_____

_____

3. What is a placebo?

_____

_____

_____

4. What are the benefits and risks of participating in a clinical trial?

_____

_____

_____

Using the following Internet link, investigate a CAM clinical trial being conducted by the National Institutes of Health. Then provide the missing information in Table 27-3.

http://nccam.nih.gov/research/clinicaltrials/alltrials.htm

TABLE 27-3 Clinical Trial

Description of the study	
Eligibility criteria for participants	
Length of the study	
Location of organization or parties completing the study	
Domain of CAM	

Write a paragraph describing the clinical trial. Include the purpose (intended outcome), supporting data, and your evaluation of the method being studied.

_____

_____

_____

_____

_____

_____

_____

_____

_____

_____

_____

_____

_____

_____

_____

Education and Career Research

Use the following links, other Internet resources, and information available by telephone or mail inquiry to determine the educational cost of one complementary and alternative career and the salary that might be earned in the local area. Use the information to complete Table 27-4.

Suggested Websites

Salary.com: http://salary.com
Monster.com: http://monster.com
Occupational Outlook Handbook: http://www.bls.gov/oco/
American Chiropractic Association: http://www.acatoday.org/
American Association of Naturopathic Physicians (AANP): http://www.naturopathic.org/
National Center for Complementary and Alternative Medicine (NCCAM): http://nccam.nih.gov/

TABLE 27-4 Education and Career Research

CAREER	INSTITUTION FOR EDUCATION	COST OF EDUCATION	POTENTIAL EARNINGS

28 Veterinary Careers

VAPID VOCABULARY

Complete the crossword puzzle using the Key Terms.

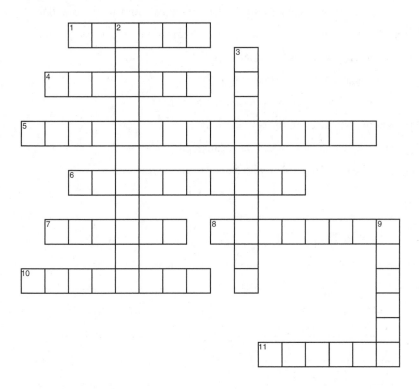

ACROSS

1 Pertaining to cattle
4 Dead body of an animal
5 Branch of veterinary medicine dealing with reproduction
6 Period of detention or isolation as a result of a disease suspected to be communicable
7 Pertaining to dogs
8 Plant or animal that lives on or within another living organism at the expense of the host organism
10 Secure against a particular disease
11 Pertaining to cats

DOWN

2 Introduction of a microorganism that has been made harmless into a human or animal for the purpose of developing immunity
3 Pertaining to animals and their diseases
9 Pertaining to horses

ABBREVIATIONS

Match each of the following abbreviations with the phrase that best describes its meaning or function. Then write the phrase or name for each of the abbreviations in the spaces provided.

Abbreviation

1. _____ AVMA
2. _____ CENSHARE
3. _____ CPR
4. _____ CVT
5. _____ DMV
6. _____ LVT
7. _____ NAVTA
8. _____ RVT
9. _____ VMD
10. _____ VT

Meaning or Function

a. Advanced treatment technique for nonresponsive animals

b. Certified health care worker who extends veterinarian duties

c. Health care worker who extends veterinarian duties with varied credentials

d. Licensed health care worker who extends veterinarian duties

e. One of two degrees for veterinarians

f. One of two degrees for veterinarians

g. Professional organization for veterinarian technicians

h. Professional organization for veterinarians

i. Program that studies human–animal relationships

j. Registered health care worker who extends veterinarian duties

1. AVMA: _____

2. CENSHARE: _____

3. CPR: _____

4. CVT: _____

5. DMV: _____

6. LVT: _____

7. NAVTA: _____

8. RVT: _____

9. VMD: _____

10. VT: _____

1. Veterinary care personnel work in a variety of settings, including _ O _ _ _ _ _ practice, O _ _ _ _ _ _ health, _ _ O _ _ _ _ _ _, zoos, and racetracks.

2. Three of the 16 recognized board specialties for veterinarians are
_ _ _ _ _ _ _ _ _ _ _ O _ _ _ _, ophthalmology, and _ _ _ medicine.

3. Three out of four veterinarians work in private practice with either _ _ _ _ _ or _ _ _ _ _ _ animals.

4. _ _ _ _ _ _ _ _ or marine biologists study plant and animal life in saltwater environments.

5. Common pets include dogs, cats, turtles, O _ _ _ _, fish, small _ _ O _ _ _ _, horses, and O _ _ _ _ _.

6. _ _ O _ _ _ _ _ _ is the process of surgical sterilization to prevent unwanted births.

7. Induction of death in a sick, severely injured, or unwanted animal is called _ _ _ _ _ _ _ _ O _ _.

8. _ O _ _ _ _ _ _ _ _ for physically and mentally ill people is rapidly becoming an accepted treatment method in many health care settings.

9. More than 150 diseases called _ _ _ _ _ _ O _ can be transmitted from animals to humans.

10. Some indications that an animal is sick include abnormal behavior, especially sudden
_ _ _ _ O _ _ _ _ _ _ _ or O _ _ _ _ _ _ _ _ _ _ _ _, abnormal discharge from any body opening.

Use the circled letters to form the answer to this jumble. Clue: What is one vital sign that may be lowered as a benefit of pet therapy?

_ _ _ _ _ _ _ _ _ _ _ _ _ _

CONCEPT APPLICATIONS

Identifying Animal Restraints
Use Figure 28-7 of the textbook to label the diagram of the animal restraints in Figure 28-1.

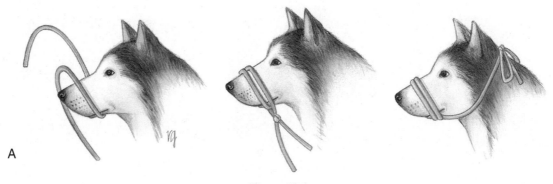

A

Figure 28-1

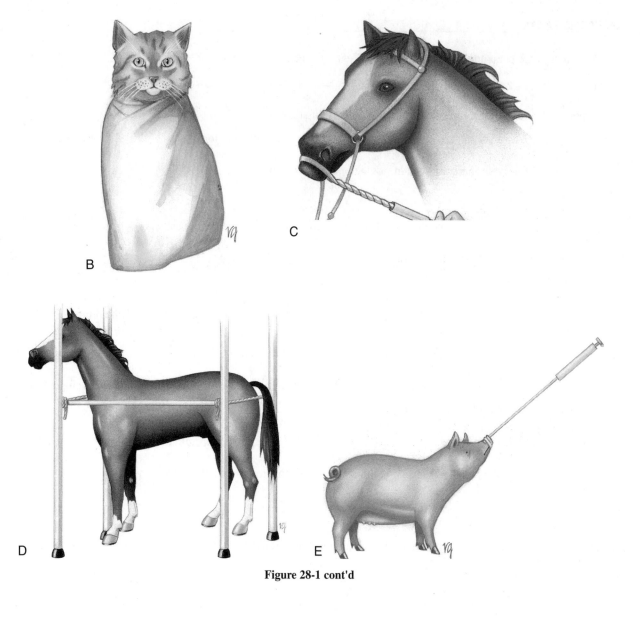

Figure 28-1 cont'd

A. _____   D. _____

B. _____   E. _____

C. _____

Identifying Sites for Blood Collection

Use Figure 28-8 in the textbook to label the diagram of the blood collection sites in Figure 28-2.

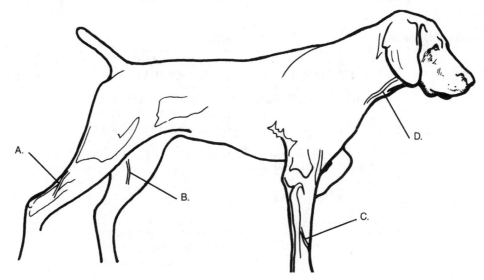

Figure 28-2

A. _____ C. _____

B. _____ D. _____

Identifying Disorders of Animals

Use the textbook to provide the missing information about animal disorders in Table 28-1. Note the name of the disorder, etiology (causing factor), signs and symptoms, and treatment and method of prevention (if any).

TABLE 28-1 Animal Disorders

DISORDER	ETIOLOGY	SIGNS AND SYMPTOMS	TREATMENT AND PREVENTION
	Virus found in fecal waste	Affects dogs, depression, loss of appetite, feces light or yellow-gray with blood	
	Feeding mismanagement, worms		
		Affects cats, symptoms vary greatly, decrease in WBC, depression, loss of appetite, dehydration	
		Affects cats, painful, frequent urination, blood in urine, depression, death	
		Affects dogs, cough, fever, gagging, loss of appetite	Self-limiting, antibiotics if bronchopneumonia develops
	Virus transmitted in saliva		
	Microorganisms transferred by dairy equipment		

Applying Your Knowledge

1. The animal disorder that can be found in humans as well as animals and is usually fatal is called _____

_____.

2. The disorder that appears in calves and is caused by bacteria in a soiled environment is called _____

_____.

3. The viral infection affecting cats that involves inflammation of the nose and trachea is called _____

_____.

4. The condition that affects dogs and is transmitted by mosquitoes is called _____

_____.

5. The condition that may occur in horses when they lick flies from their hair is called _____

_____.

Animal Health Careers

Animal Health Skills and Qualities

List three personal qualities and skills that are important in animal health careers.

1. _____

2. _____

3. _____

Identifying Animal Health Careers

Use the textbook to provide the missing information about animal health careers in Table 28-2.

TABLE 28-2 Animal Health Careers

CAREER TITLE	YEARS OF EDUCATION	DESCRIPTION OF JOB DUTIES AND OPPORTUNITIES	CREDENTIALS REQUIRED
		Research on ocean life; work in ecology; usually employed by universities, private industry or the government	
			DVM or VMD, licensed by the state
		Research, food inspection, laboratory or private clinic; prepare and test vaccines, collect specimens, administer medication	
	On-the-job training or home study		
		Use genetic traits to meet breeding needs of owners	

Applying Your Knowledge

1. The professional who might specialize in practice with small or large animals is the _____.

2. Extended duties, such as teeth cleaning, removal of sutures, and administration of intravenous fluids, may be learned by the _____.

3. To obtain a cow that produces more milk, the dairy farmer may consult an _____.

4. Environmental conditions such as soil and water salinity and temperature may be studied by the

_____.

Performing an Animal Health Assessment

Read all of the instructions before beginning this activity. Laboratory activities should be completed under the supervision of a qualified professional only.

Equipment and Supplies

Domestic animal, such as a cat or dog
Stethoscope

Directions

1. Maintain medical asepsis by practicing frequent handwashing when handling animals.
2. Restrain the animal as needed to prevent injury to yourself or to the animal.
3. Observe the animal to complete the assessment form in Figure 28-3. Use caution to avoid injury to yourself or to the animal.
4. Complete the temperature assessment and anal sac examination under the supervision of a qualified animal care professional only.
5. Release and reward the animal with affection.
6. Clean the equipment and return it to the designated location.

Pet's name: _____

Owner's name: _____

Species: _____ Breed: _____

Sex: ____ Age: ____ Weight _____ Temp: _____

Exam date: _____ By: _____

Examination Checklist

Coat and Skin

___ Appear normal   ___ Matted
___ Dull   ___ Tumors

Coat and Skin (cont.)

___ Scaly   ___ Itchy
___ Dry   ___ Parasites
___ Oily   ___ Other_____
___ Shedding   _____

Recommendation: _____

Eyes

___ Appear normal   ___ Infection
___ Discharge   ___ Cataract ___ L ___ R
___ Inflamed   ___ Other_____
___ Eyelid deformity   _____

Recommendation: _____

Figure 28-3

Drawing Conclusions

1. Describe any abnormal findings from the assessment. What might be the cause of the abnormality, if one is found?

_____

_____

_____

CRITICAL THINKING

Animal Rights

Most scientists believe that research that uses animals is necessary to develop new treatments and drugs and to understand human behavior. Some people who care about the welfare of animals believe that research could be completed without using animals. The controversy also involves the use of animals for making fur coats and for testing cosmetics. More than 90% of the animals used in research are bred for that purpose.

Guidelines for laboratories that use animals in research have been developed by the National Institutes of Health (NIH). The laboratory must provide the NIH with written documentation to show the designs of the experiments. It must also document other work in the same field to show that the tests do not duplicate other studies. The laboratory administration must pledge that animals used for research will not experience unnecessary pain without anesthesia.

Examining the Evidence

1. Which animal health care professional might be the best person to determine what is considered to be "humane care"? Explain your answer.

_____

_____

_____

2. Why do you support or not support the use of animals for research purposes?

_____

_____

_____

3. Why do or do you not believe that the guidelines used by the NIH to regulate research laboratories are adequate?

_____

_____

_____

Prove It!

Owning a pet has been found to have many beneficial effects. Some of these benefits for pet owners include lowering of their blood pressure, protection, and assistance with activities of daily living. The manner in which people treat their pets has also been a subject of research. For example, some people treat their pet as a member of the family, buying presents, preparing and feeding them table food, and so forth. Another area of interest is the manner in which people speak to pets. Some address their pets with gestures as much as or more than words, others are authoritative, and still others speak in "baby talk."

Use the preceding information for ideas to design an experiment that will determine a characteristic of the relationship between people and their pets. Conduct the experiment and report the results to the class.

Chapter **28** **Veterinary Careers**

Examining the Evidence

1. What is the hypothesis of your experiment?

_____

_____

_____

2. Describe the design of your experiment, including materials and time limits.

_____

_____

_____

3. What is the controlled variable in your experiment?

_____

_____

_____

4. What is the variable in your experiment?

_____

_____

_____

5. What conclusion were you able to draw regarding your hypothesis?

_____

_____

_____

INTERNET ACTIVITIES

Education and Career Research

Use the following links, other Internet resources, and information available by telephone or mail inquiry to determine the educational cost of one veterinary career and the salary that might be earned in the local area. Use the information to complete Table 28-3.

Suggested Websites

Salary.com: http://salary.com
Monster.com: http://monster.com
Occupational Outlook Handbook: http://www.bls.gov/oco/
American Veterinary Medical Association: http://www.avma.org/
National Association of Veterinary Technicians in America (NAVTA): http://www.navta.net/

TABLE 28-3 Education and Career Research

CAREER	INSTITUTION FOR EDUCATION	COST OF EDUCATION	POTENTIAL EARNINGS

29 Community and Social Careers

VAPID VOCABULARY

Complete the crossword puzzle using the Key Terms.

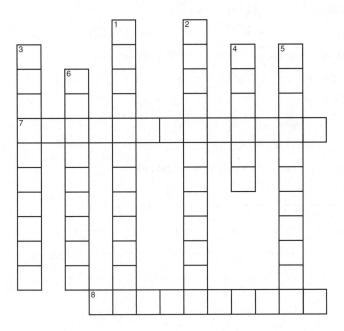

ACROSS

7 Sensory perception that occurs in waking state but does not have external stimulus
8 Addiction to drugs or alcohol

DOWN

1 Capable of being transmitted from one person or animal to another
2 Process of becoming secure against a particular disease or pathogen
3 Unpleasant symptoms resulting with stoppage of drugs or substances on which a person is dependent; symptoms include anxiety, insomnia, irritability, impaired attention, and physical illness
4 Carrier that transfers an infective agent from one host to another
5 Pertaining to the study of people as a group, especially of statistical groupings according to age, gender, and environmental factors
6 Condition of being defiled or impure

Chapter **29** **Community and Social Careers**

Copyright © 2012, 2007, 2003, 1997, 1990 by Mosby, Inc., an affiliate of Elsevier Inc. All rights reserved.

ABBREVIATIONS

Match each of the following abbreviations with the phrase that best describes its meaning or function. Then write the phrase or name for each of the abbreviations in the spaces provided.

Abbreviation	Meaning or Function
1. _____ AAOHN	a. Child care specialist who is certified
2. _____ BSW	b. Main organization for public health at the federal level
3. _____ CCLS	c. Organization that certifies child life professionals
4. _____ CDC	d. Organization that collects statistical information about populations
5. _____ CLC	e. Professional organization for occupational health nurses
6. _____ DSW	f. Professional organization for social workers
7. _____ GSW	g. Risk survey of teenagers
8. _____ HHS	h. Social worker who completes 4 years of university
9. _____ NASW	i. Social worker who completes 6 years or more of university
10. _____ YRBSS	j. Social worker who specializes in working with the elderly

1. AAOHN: _____

2. BSW: _____

3. CCLS: _____

4. CDC: _____

5. CLC: _____

6. DSW: _____

7. GSW: _____

8. HHS: _____

9. NASW: _____

10. YRBSS: _____

1. Community and social health care have broad goals and focus on the health needs of

   a _ _ _ _ _ _ _ Ⓞ _ _.

2. The community and social health care Ⓞ _ _ _ _ _ is involved in the search for the source

   of _ _ _ _ _ _ _ and the use of technical and regulatory means to protect the population from

   environmental, social, and behavioral hazards.

3. _ _ _ _ Ⓞ _ _ _ _ _ _ _ _ _ _ _ _ _ identify and explain the social

   factors affecting the care of patients.

4. _ _ _ _ _ _ _ _ _ _ _ _ _ _ _ _ Ⓞ _ _ _ _ _ _ specialize

   in providing assistance to the elderly.

5. The three levels of education for professional social workers are the bachelor's degree, the master's degree, and

   the _ _ _ _ _ _ _ _ degree.

6. _ _ _ _ _ _ _ _ _ _ help their patients solve problems of personal, social, career, and

   educational development.

7. The _ _ _ _ _ _ _ _ _ _ _ _ _ _ _ Ⓞ _ _ _ _ works in health care

   settings and focuses on the emotional and developmental needs of children.

8. Drug dependence is the _ Ⓞ _ _ _ _ _ _ or _ _ _ _ _ _ _ _ _ _ _ _ _ _ Ⓞ _

   need to continue taking a drug.

9. _ _ _ _ _ Ⓞ _ _ _ _ may be used to increase the activity of the central nervous system, whereas

   Ⓞ _ _ _ _ _ _ _ _ _ _ _ have the opposite effect.

10. Two drugs commonly associated with "_ _ _ _ Ⓞ _ _ _" are flunitrazepam and gamma

    hydroxybutyrate.

   Use the circled letters to form the answer to this jumble. Clue: What is the physical reaction to stopping a drug that has caused dependence called?

   _ _ _ _ _ _ _ _ _ _ _

Community and Social Health Careers

Community and Social Health Skills and Qualities

List three personal qualities and skills that are important in community and social health careers.

1. _____

2. _____

3. _____

Identifying Community and Social Health Careers

Use the textbook to provide the missing information about community and social health careers in Table 29-1.

TABLE 29-1 Community and Social Careers

CAREER TITLE	YEARS OF EDUCATION	DESCRIPTION OF JOB DUTIES AND OPPORTUNITIES	CREDENTIALS REQUIRED
			MS, most states require licensure
		Determines suitability of foster homes and adoption applicants	
		Provides daily care for children in institutions under supervision	
		Completes applications for unemployment, food stamps, and other services	
			BSW, MSW, DSW, ACSW

Applying Your Knowledge

1. The health practitioner who assists children who are confined to the hospital with play therapy may be educated as

   a _____.

2. Counselors who specialize in career opportunities and learning a trade are called _____.

3. A disabled child might be assisted while attending school by the _____.

4. Schools, rehabilitation agencies, mental health or correctional facilities, and colleges are just a few of the settings in

   which _____ work.

5. Counselors who specialize in substance abuse may be educated as _____

   or _____.

Observing the Spread of Microorganisms

Read all of the directions before beginning the activity. Work in groups of six or seven for this activity. Laboratory activities should be completed under the supervision of a qualified professional only.

Equipment and Supplies

6 to 8 applicators
Autoclave or bleach
Beaker of warm water
Grease pencil or china marker
Incubator
Package of dry yeast
1 peppermint candy
3 potato dextrose agar plates per group

Directions

1. Practice good medical asepsis by using frequent handwashing technique.
2. Use the skills listed in the textbook to prepare a sterile plate of potato dextrose agar.
3. Use a grease pencil to draw a line on the outside of each plate to divide the agar plate into halves or fourths, as directed by the instructor. There should be one section of the plate for each student in the group.
4. Number each section of the plate consecutively to eight with the grease pencil.
5. Prepare a solution of warm water and baking yeast in a beaker.
6. Soak a piece of hard peppermint candy in the beaker for 3 to 5 minutes.
7. While the candy is soaking, all students in the group should wash their hands thoroughly with warm water and soap. Rinse completely.
8. Designate each student of the group by a number that corresponds to one of the agar plate sections.
9. Student #1 should remove the candy from the beaker and rub it in the palm of his or her right hand. Then the candy is discarded in an appropriate waste receptacle.
10. Student #1 shakes hands with student #2. Participants should not touch any surface with their hands after shaking hands with the previous student of the group until the culture is taken from the hand.
11. Student #2 shakes hands with student #3.
12. Student #3 shakes hands with student #4, and so forth to student #6 or #7. It is important that the handshaking be done rapidly down the line of students.
13. During the process of handshaking, the last student should "culture" the palm of student #1 and streak section #1 of the plate with the specimen gathered. Student #1 may then wash his or her hands.
14. After student #1's culture is done, that student may culture student #2's palm and streak the section labeled #2 with the specimen.
15. After student #2's culture is done, the hands may be washed, and that student may culture student #3's palm and streak the plate.
16. The procedure is continued until all students' palms have been cultured and plate sections have been streaked for each.
17. After the culturing is done, incubate the plates upside down at approximately 37° C for 24 hours. Observe the plates and record any growth that occurs.
18. Continue incubation and observation every day for 5 days.
19. Sterilize or disinfect the agar plates before discarding them.

Drawing Conclusions

1. What type of organism was cultured on the potato dextrose agar? Did any other organisms grow on the plates?

_____

_____

_____

2. In which section did growth occur first?

_____

_____

_____

3. In which section was the growth the heaviest?

_____

_____

_____

4. In which section was the growth the lightest?

_____

_____

_____

5. How was the organism transferred from student #1 to student #7?

_____

_____

_____

6. Why were all of the students' hands washed before the activity was started?

_____

_____

_____

7. Why did the plates not contain growth of many types of organisms?

_____

_____

_____

8. Why is 37° C used for incubation of microorganisms?

_____

_____

_____

CRITICAL THINKING

Unsolved Mysteries

This activity is adapted from the VQI (Vector Quest 1) series developed by the Iowa Medical Foundation. It allows you to be an epidemiologist, or medical detective. Use the information to answer the following questions.

Situation One

Farmington, Iowa is experiencing an increased rate of cancer cases and a resulting increase in deaths. The residents speculate about the power lines, old tanneries, the water, the air, and genetics. Any number of reasons, including chance, might explain this cluster.

Examining the Evidence

1. What variables might be considered in determining a solution to this mystery?

_____

_____

_____

2. What questions would you like answered to help you determine the source of this cluster of illnesses?

_____

_____

_____

3. Describe how information could be obtained or an experiment performed to determine the source of this cluster.

_____

_____

_____

4. Can you think of any health measures that might be recommended to the population of Farmington to limit their risk of developing this cancer?

_____

_____

_____

Situation Two

In the Northwest, Alaska Airlines has identified a particular plane that has a history of "making people sick."

Examining the Evidence

1. What variables might be considered in determining a solution to this mystery?

_____

_____

_____

2. What questions would you like answered to help you determine the source of this cluster of illnesses?

_____

_____

_____

3. Describe how information could be obtained or an experiment performed to determine the source of this cluster.

_____

_____

_____

4. Can you think of any health measures that might be recommended to the airline to limit passengers' risk of developing this disease?

_____

_____

_____

Excite

Epidemiology in the Classroom

Use the following link to complete the CDC Excite online epidemiology activity. Review the incidents and answer the questions about epidemiology.

http://www.cdc.gov/excite/classroom/intro_epi.htm

Questions

1. Describe each of the following types of epidemiology design studies:

   Cross-sectional— _____

   _____

   _____

   Cohort— _____

   _____

   _____

   Case control— _____

   _____

   _____

2. Describe why one of the methods might be better than the others to study each of the unsolved mystery cases.

   Situation One— _____

   _____

   _____

   Situation Two— _____

   _____

   _____

Education and Career Research

Use the following links, other Internet resources, and information available by telephone or mail inquiry to determine the educational cost of one community and social health career and the salary that might be earned in the local area. Use the information to complete Table 29-2.

Suggested Websites

Salary.com: http://salary.com
Monster.com: http://monster.com
Occupational Outlook Handbook: http://www.bls.gov/oco/
American Association of Occupational Health Nursing (AAOHN): https://www.aaohn.org/
National Association of Social Workers (NASW): http://www.socialworkers.org/

TABLE 29-2 Education and Career Research

CAREER	INSTITUTION FOR EDUCATION	COST OF EDUCATION	POTENTIAL EARNINGS

VAPID VOCABULARY

Complete the crossword puzzle using the Key Terms.

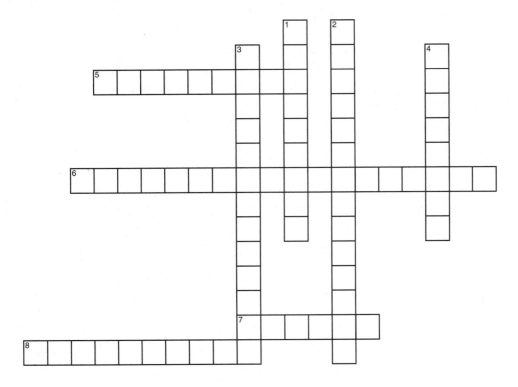

ACROSS

5 Major mental disorder in which the individual loses contact with reality
6 Awareness of position in relation to time, space, and person (Two words)
7 Persistent abnormal dread or fear
8 Study of human and animal behavior, normal and abnormal

DOWN

1 Physical confinement
2 Functional disturbance of the mind in which the individual is aware that reactions are not normal
3 Treatment of discomfort, dysfunction, or diseases by methods designed to understand and cope with problems
4 Conduct, actions that can be observed

ABBREVIATIONS

Match each of the following abbreviations with the phrase that best describes its meaning or function. Then write the phrase or name for each of the abbreviations in the spaces provided.

Abbreviation

1. _____ APA
2. _____ APNA
3. _____ EdD
4. _____ LOC
5. _____ NCHSE
6. _____ NIMH
7. _____ OJT
8. _____ PhD
9. _____ PsyD
10. _____ RO

Meaning or Function

a. Description of orientation
b. Doctorate degree in education
c. Doctorate degree in philosophy
d. Doctorate degree in psychology
e. Learning while working
f. Method to maintain and improve level of consciousness
g. National organization for mental health
h. Organization that certifies mental health technicians
i. Professional organization for psychiatrists
j. Professional organizations for psychiatric nurses

1. APA: _____

2. APNA: _____

3. EdD: _____

4. LOC: _____

5. NCHSE: _____

6. NIMH: _____

7. OJT: _____

8. PhD: _____

9. PsyD: _____

10. RO: _____

JUST THE FACTS

1. The function of the mental health care team is to provide care and treatment for individuals with disorders of the
_ _ _ Ọ, _ _ _ _ _ _ _ _, or _ _ _ _ _ _ _ _ Ọ.

2. It is now commonly accepted that a person's emotional and mental states may either cause or have some effect on all _ _ _ _ _ Ọ _ _ disorders.

3. _ _ _ _ _ _ _ Ọ _ _ _ _ _ _ are licensed physicians specializing in the treatment of mental, emotional, and behavioral disorders.

4. _ _ _ _ _ _ _ Ọ _ _ _ _ _ _ are professionals, not physicians, who specialize in the treatment of mental and emotional disorders.

5. _ _ _ _ _ _ _ _ _ _ _ _ _ is a state of mind in which a person can cope with problems and maintain emotional balance and satisfaction in living.

6. __ __ __ __ __ __ Ⓞ __ __ __ __ __ __ __ are functional disturbances of the mind.

7. __ __ __ __ __ __ __ __ __ __ are severe or major mental disorders in which the individual is not in contact with reality.

8. Mental __ __ __ __ Ⓞ __ __ includes the methods used to preserve and promote mental health.

9. Loss of __ __ __ __ __ __ __ __ __ __ __ __ may result from loss of hearing, sight, or confinement.

10. Use of __ __ __ __ __ Ⓞ __ __ __ __ must be ordered by a physician and only after proper instruction has been given for its use.

Use the circled letters to form the answer to this jumble. Clue: What is a useful tool in helping a patient maintain reality orientation?

__ __ __ __ __ __ __ __

CONCEPT APPLICATIONS

Recognizing Substance Abuse

List 10 signs and symptoms that might indicate substance abuse.

1. _____

2. _____

3. _____

4. _____

5. _____

6. _____

7. _____

8. _____

9. _____

10. _____

Applying Your Knowledge

1. Which of the signs and symptoms you have listed might result from causes other than substance abuse?

_____

_____

_____

2. What type of intervention could you use with a person showing the signs and symptoms you have listed to determine whether substance abuse is the cause?

_____

_____

_____

3. What would you do if you were concerned that a friend might be using mind-altering substances?

_____

_____

_____

4. What resources are available in the community to help an individual with substance abuse problems?

_____

_____

_____

Identifying Mental Messages

Psychosocial health care professionals often use the concept of "self-talk" in helping people deal with emotional concerns. Each person receives many positive and negative messages from others and themselves every day. Complete Table 30-1 by changing the negative message to one that is positive. Add five negative messages that you give yourself or that someone else gives you. Change the negative message into one that is positive.

TABLE 30-1 Mental Messages

	MESSAGE—NEGATIVE	MESSAGE—POSITIVE
Example	I am (you are) always late. I (you) can't ever get a B in math. I'm (you're) so fat. I (you) never get along with him/her. I'm (you're) such a slob.	I have a tendency to be late, but with better planning, I can arrive on time.

Mental Health Careers

Mental Health Skills and Qualities

List three personal qualities and skills that are important in mental health careers.

1. _____

2. _____

3. _____

Identifying Mental Health Careers

Use the textbook to provide the missing information about mental health careers in Table 30-2.

TABLE 30-2 Mental Health Careers

CAREER TITLE	YEARS OF EDUCATION	DESCRIPTION OF JOB DUTIES AND OPPORTUNITIES	CREDENTIALS REQUIRED
			PhD, EdD, or PsyD
		Interview, lead group sessions, give daily care, make home visits, in some states may administer medications	
		Treatment of mental, emotional, and behavioral disorders, may prescribe medications	
	4- to 6-month program or on-the-job training		

Applying Your Knowledge

1. For treatment of a mental disorder that requires medication, the client would probably seek the care of a

   _____ .

2. Assistance with activities of daily living, such as reality orientation, would probably be accomplished by the

   _____ working under the supervision of the professional.

3. In some states the health care worker called the _____ is also called a mental

   health associate or human service worker.

4. The professional who uses interviews, testing, and observation to treat mental disorders but who does not prescribe

   medication is called a _____ .

5. The mental health specialist who practices in diverse areas of clinical, quantitative, consumer, environmental, and

   organizational behavior is probably a _____ .

CRITICAL THINKING

Mental Health Stigma

Most people who suffer from mental disorders recover completely and live active and productive lives. Understanding and treatment of the mentally ill have evolved from placing the individual with a mental disorder in an asylum to allowing the person active participation in society.

However, a stigma (or attitude) still exists in society that people with mental disorders are weak or violent. Some people believe that all mentally ill people should be "locked up" and kept away from others.

In the 1970s a man was considered by a political party to run for vice president of the United States. The man led an active and complete life. He had a family and had done many great things in his community and political party. However, when it became known that he had been treated at one time for a mental disorder, the party dropped his name from the ticket.

1. Why do some people believe that people with mental illnesses are weak or violent?

_____

_____

_____

2. When should limitations be placed on the activities of a person with a mental disorder?

_____

_____

_____

3. For what kind of disorder do you believe that a mentally ill person should be refused a driver's license?

_____

_____

_____

4. How might the political party's decision to drop the candidate from its ticket affect another person who suffers from depression or other mental disorders but who wants to run for political office in the future?

_____

_____

_____

What's "News"?

In 1994, researchers reported the results of studies on human psychosocial behavior, some of which were controversial. Respond to each of the following conclusions that researchers drew from their studies. Use examples from your own experiences or information you have learned to agree or disagree with the research conclusions.

Psychologists reported that memories of stressful and emotional events are retained longer due to the release of hormones.

Response:

_____

_____

_____

A study using rhesus monkeys found that certain behaviors keep aggression in control in crowded conditions.
Response:

_____

_____

_____

Researchers determined that babies babble with acoustic structure and patterns of speech at 2 months of age. Others concluded that babies recognize their name at 4½ months of age.
Response:

_____

_____

_____

In 1998 a paper in a medical journal linked autism to vaccines, particularly the MMR. In 2010, the article was retracted by the magazine citing faulty research techniques that included a study group of only 12 children chosen from children attending the birthday party of the researcher's own child.

Response:

_____

_____

_____

INTERNET ACTIVITIES

Education and Career Research

Use the following links, other Internet resources, and information available by telephone or mail inquiry to determine the educational cost of one mental health career and the salary that might be earned in the local area. Use the information to complete Table 30-3.

Suggested Websites

Salary.com: http://salary.com
Monster.com: http://monster.com
Occupational Outlook Handbook: http://www.bls.gov/oco/
American Psychology Association (APA): http://www.apa.org/
American Psychiatric Nurses Association (APNA): http://www.apna.org/i4a/pages/index.cfm?pageid=1

TABLE 30-3 Education and Career Research

CAREER	INSTITUTION FOR EDUCATION	COST OF EDUCATION	POTENTIAL EARNINGS

VAPID VOCABULARY

Complete the crossword puzzle using the Key Terms.

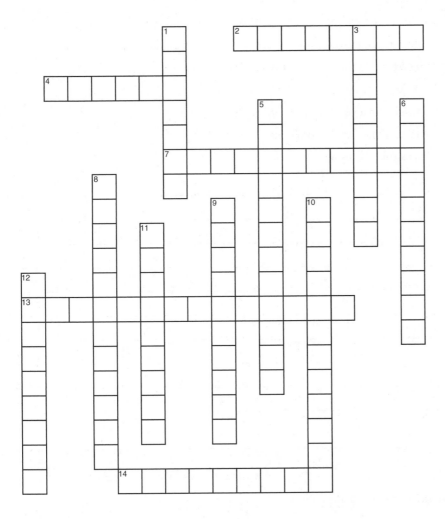

ACROSS

2 Prepare, package, compound, or label for delivery according to a lawful order of a qualified practitioner
4 Regulation of size, frequency, and amount of medication
7 Art or science of custom design, fabrication, and fitting of artificial limbs
13 Restoration of normal form and function after injury or illness
14 Number of times an event occurs in a given period; measured in cycles per second (hertz [Hz]) in hearing

DOWN

1 Treatment of disease; science and art of healing
3 Device used to deliver a spray or mist of medication into the lungs
5 Enunciation of words and syllables, how sounds are spoken
6 Lack of ability to function in the manner that most people function physically or mentally
8 Study of the actions and uses of drugs
9 Artificial device applied to replace a partially or totally missing body part
10 Application of water
11 Science of hearing
12 Art or science of custom designing, fabrication, and fitting of braces

ABBREVIATIONS

Match each of the following abbreviations with the phrase that best describes its meaning or function. Then write the phrase or name for each of the abbreviations in the spaces provided.

Abbreviation	Meaning or Function
1. _____ ADT	a. Educational degree for pharmacists
2. _____ AOPA	b. Examination that compares similar sounding words
3. _____ COTA	c. Health care worker who runs a heart-lung machine
4. _____ ECT	d. Health care worker who helps patients reach independence
5. _____ OTC	e. Health care worker who restores function and relieves pain
6. _____ OT	f. Health care worker who treats pulmonary conditions
7. _____ PharmD	g. Medications that do not require a prescription
8. _____ PDR	h. Organization that certifies occupational therapists
9. _____ PT	i. Organization that certifies orthotists
10. _____ RT	j. Reference for drug usage

1. ADT: _____

2. AOPA: _____

3. COTA: _____

4. ECT: _____

5. OTC: _____

6. OT: _____

7. PharmD: _____

8. PDR: _____

9. PT: _____

10. RT: _____

JUST THE FACTS

1. The _ _ _ _ _ _ _ _ _ _ _ _ _ _ ◯ team provides services designed to overcome physical, developmental, behavioral, or emotional disabilities.

2. _ _ _ _ _ _ _ ◯ _ therapists work to restore function, relieve pain, and prevent _ _ _ _ _ _ _ _ _ _ _ after disease, injury, or loss of a body part.

3. _ _ ◯ _ _ _ _ _ _ _ _ _ _ _ _ _ _ _ help patients strengthen and coordinate body movements using exercise.

4. _ _ _ _ _ _ _ _ _ _ _ modify and provide footwear to patients with imperfectly formed feet.

5. _ _ _ _ ◯ _ _ _ _ _ _ ◯ _ therapy helps patients reach the highest level of independent living by overcoming physical injury, birth defects, aging, or emotional and developmental problems.

Chapter **31** **Rehabilitative Careers**

6. __ __ __ Ⓞ __ __ __ __ __   __ __ __ __ Ⓞ __ __ __ work under the supervision of the team physician in a variety of amateur and professional sports and other settings.

7. __ __ __ __ __ __ __ __ __ __ __ Ⓞ mix and dispense drugs according to prescriptions written by physicians, veterinarians, dentists, and other authorized professionals.

8. __ __ __ __ __ __ __ Ⓞ __ __ __ __ therapists evaluate the patient to administer respiratory care and operate life support equipment under the supervision of a physician.

9. __ __ __ __ __ __ __ __ __ Ⓞ __ __ __ is the study of drugs, their actions, dosages, side effects, indications, and contraindications.

10. __ __ Ⓞ __ and Ⓞ __ __ __ __ applications are used in physical therapy to allow increased movement of joints.

Use the circled letters to form the answer to this jumble. Clue: What is one of three common methods used to administer oxygen?

__ __ __ __ __   __ __ __ __ __ __ __

CONCEPT APPLICATIONS

Comparing Fluid Measurements

Three systems are currently used to measure fluid volumes: the SI (or metric), apothecary, and household systems. The metric system, developed in France, is used internationally and is based on the decimal system, using units of 10. The apothecary system was the original system used in the United States by pharmacists. The household system was developed for use with common items found in the home. Study the chart of approximate equivalents to answer the questions.

METRIC	APOTHECARY	HOUSEHOLD
1000 mL	32 oz	1 qt
500 mL	16 oz	1 pt
30 mL	1 oz	2 T
4 mL	1 dr	1 tsp
0.06 mL	1 min	1 gt

KEY TO SYMBOLS

cc = cubic centimeter
mL = milliliter
oz = fluid ounce (℥)
dr = fluid dram (ℨ)
min = fluid minim (℧)
qt = quart
pt = pint
T = tablespoon
tsp = teaspoon
gt = drop

Applying Your Knowledge

1. How many ounces are equivalent to 60 cc?

_____

2. How many drops are equivalent to 1 teaspoon?

_____

3. How many cubic centimeters are equivalent to 10 ounces?

_____

4. How many liters are equivalent to 1200 cc?

_____

5. Which system is most easily changed from one unit of measurement to another in the same system?

_____

Calculating Drug Dosages

Use Table 31-4 of the textbook to calculate the following dosage problems.

Applying Your Knowledge

1. The order is to give the client a medication at the dosage of 10 mL every hour. What would the correct dosage be in teaspoons?

_____

2. The order is to give the client a medication at the dosage of 300 mg. You have tablets that are 500 mg strength. How many tablets would you need to give the client for a correct dosage?

_____

3. The order is to give the client a medication at the dosage of 15 mg/kg of weight, three times a day. You have a dosage of grains. The client weighs 120 pounds. How much of the medication do you need to have on hand for a 24-hour period?

_____

Using the Manual Alphabet

Use Figure 31-6 of the textbook to decode the message in Figure 31-1. Construct a message of your own. Practice "signing" the message with a partner.

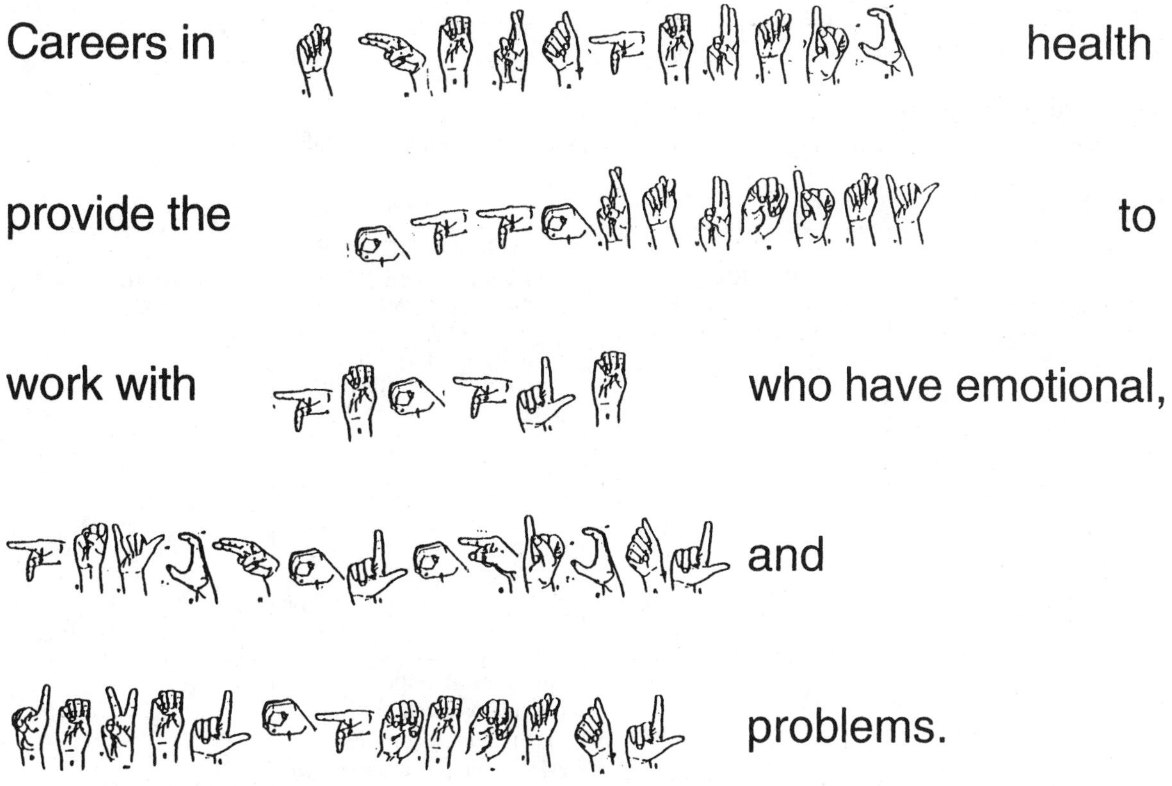

Careers in [sign language illustration] health

provide the [sign language illustration] to

work with [sign language illustration] who have emotional,

[sign language illustration] and

[sign language illustration] problems.

Figure 31-1

Applying Your Knowledge

1. What does the message say?

_____

_____

_____

2. Why would it be preferable to some hearing-impaired individuals to use signs that indicate words rather than letters?

_____

_____

_____

3. Approximately 10% of the parents of hearing-impaired individuals learn to sign. Why might this be true?

_____

_____

_____

Rehabilitative Careers

Rehabilitative Skills and Qualities

List three personal qualities and skills that are important in rehabilitative careers.

1. _____

2. _____

3. _____

Identifying Rehabilitative Careers

Use the textbook to provide the missing information about rehabilitative careers in Table 31-1.

TABLE 31-1 Rehabilitative Careers

CAREER TITLE	YEARS OF EDUCATION	DESCRIPTION OF JOB DUTIES AND OPPORTUNITIES	CREDENTIALS REQUIRED
		Design, fabricate, and fit braces and strengthening devices	
			BS; MS preferred; licensed by the state
		Analyzes activities to provide assistance to disabled to accomplish ADLs, plan, and supervise programs	
			PharmD or BS Pharm

CRITICAL THINKING

Care of Hearing Aids

Hearing aids are devices that act as miniature loudspeakers to make sounds louder. The hearing aid does not cure the hearing impairment. It requires proper care and maintenance to be effective. Hearing aids may be worn:

- In the ear
- Behind the ear
- Behind the ear with a plastic tube leading into the ear canal
- Built into eyeglasses
- Clipped to the wearer's clothing with a cord and button-like receiver in the ear

The following are simple guidelines to use when speaking to an individual wearing a hearing aid, as well as steps for care of the hearing aid.

- Face the person directly when speaking.
- Speak clearly, slowly, and naturally.
- Do not place the hearing aid in direct sunlight or on hot surfaces.
- Do not use hair spray while the hearing aid is in place.
- Do not get the hearing aid wet.
- Clean the ear mold by carefully removing wax with a pipe cleaner or toothpick.
- Wash the ear mold in mild soap and water if it can be detached from the hearing aid.
- Inspect the tubing for cracks, loose connections, and twisting, which may indicate the need for replacement.

346

Examining the Evidence

1. Would it be necessary to speak loudly to a person wearing a hearing aid?

_____

_____

_____

2. Why is it important to remove the hearing aid before taking a shower or bath?

_____

_____

_____

3. Rubbing alcohol has the property of drying materials. Why is it important to avoid the use of it when cleaning hearing aids?

_____

_____

_____

Living with Disabilities

Physical disabilities affect people of every age, race, and socioeconomic status. It is estimated that up to 40 million Americans have some form of physical disability. These disabilities may be the result of stroke, head or spinal injury, arthritis, neurologic disease, or back pain. The following questions are designed to help you explore your knowledge of and attitude toward disabilities.

Examining the Evidence

1. What are three adaptations that have been made for students who use a wheelchair in your school?

_____

_____

_____

2. Are any areas of your school inaccessible to students in a wheelchair?

_____

_____

_____

3. What are three adaptive techniques that would be needed in caring for a person without sight?

_____

_____

_____

4. Do you think a disabled person would appreciate being looked at or away from when you walk past?

_____

_____

_____

5. Do you think it is a good idea to talk to a disabled person about the disability or to avoid talking about the disability?

_____

_____

_____

6. Do you think a person with limited mobility would appreciate or resent help with tasks, such as putting on a coat or lifting books?

_____

_____

_____

INTERNET ACTIVITIES

Education and Career Research

Use the following links, other Internet resources, and information available by telephone or mail inquiry to determine the educational cost of one rehabilitative career and the salary that might be earned in the local area. Use the information to complete Table 31-2.

Suggested Websites

Salary.com: http://salary.com
Monster.com: http://monster.com
Occupational Outlook Handbook: http://www.bls.gov/oco/
American Physical Therapy Association (APTA): http://apta.org
American Association for Respiratory Care (AARC): http://www.aarc.org/
National Athletic Trainers' Association (NATA): http://www.nata.org/

TABLE 31-2 Education and Career Research

CAREER	INSTITUTION FOR EDUCATION	COST OF EDUCATION	POTENTIAL EARNINGS

32 Emergency Health Careers

VAPID VOCABULARY

Complete the crossword puzzle using the Key Terms.

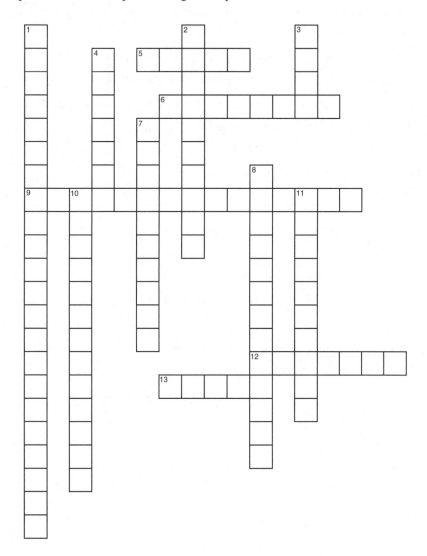

ACROSS

5 Condition of acute failure of the peripheral circulation
6 Pertaining to a crisis or danger of death
9 Pertaining to the heart and lungs
12 Sudden attack of a disease; uncontrolled muscle movements of epilepsy
13 Poison produced by animals, plants, or bacteria

DOWN

1 Placing a tube within or through the trachea (two words)
2 Instrument used to compress a blood vessel by application around an extremity
3 Subjective sensation or motor phenomenon that precedes and marks the onset of a seizure
4 Spotted, with patches of color
7 Abnormal external or internal bleeding
8 Responsiveness of the mind and to the impressions made by the senses
10 Restoration of life or consciousness of a person who is apparently dead by using artificial respiration and cardiac massage
11 Act of inhaling foreign matter, usually emesis, into the respiratory tract

349

ABBREVIATIONS

Match each of the following abbreviations with the phrase that best describes its meaning or function. Then write the phrase or name for each of the abbreviations in the spaces provided.

Abbreviation	Meaning or Function
1. _____ ACLS	a. Certified health care worker who provides advanced emergency treatment
2. _____ AED	b. Certified nurse who treats critically ill patients
3. _____ AHA	c. Electronic rescue treatment for victim of cardiac arrest
4. _____ CCRN	d. Emergency heart care
5. _____ CPR	e. Health care worker who provides care for accident victims
6. _____ DAN	f. Organization that establishes widely accepted CPR guidelines
7. _____ ECC	g. Organization that provides insurance and education for scuba diving accidents
8. _____ EMS	h. Organized group of rescue personnel and services
9. _____ EMT	i. Professional organization for EMTs
10. _____ NAEMT	j. Rescue treatment for victim of cardiac arrest

1. ACLS: _____

2. AED: _____

3. AHA: _____

4. CCRN: _____

5. CPR: _____

6. DAN: _____

7. ECC: _____

8. EMS: _____

9. EMT: _____

10. NAEMT: _____

1. The goal of modern emergency care is immediate aid, or first aid, at the __ Ⓞ __ __ __   __ __

   __ __ __ __ __ __.

2. Emergency medical technicians work under the supervision of a Ⓞ __ __ __ __ __ __ __ __ to provide

   care to the acutely ill or injured person in the prehospital setting.

3. The EMT-P, or __ __ __ __ __ __ __ __ __ __, provides advanced life support.

4. __ __ __ __ __ __ __   __ __ __ __ __ Ⓞ professions have evolved as a career opportunity with the

   use of helicopters to transport victims to emergency facilities.

5. The first priority of the rescuer is to __ __ __ __ __ __ the victim from any immediate danger and

   determine the level of __ __ Ⓞ __ __ __ __ __ __ __ __ __ __ of the victim.

6. __ __ __ __ __ is the response of the cardiovascular system to the presence of adrenalin, resulting in capillary

   constriction.

7. The severity of a burn is determined by the __ __ __ __ Ⓞ __ __ __, __ __ __ __ __ __, and

   __ __ __ __.

8. __ __ __ __ __ Ⓞ __ __ __ can be classified as closed or open.

9. Exposure to heat can result in muscle __ __ __ __ __ __ __ __, heat

   __ __ __ __ Ⓞ __ __ __ __ __, or __ __ __ __ __ __ __ __ __ __ __ __.

10. All emergency workers use substance isolation precautions to prevent the spread

    of __ __ __ Ⓞ __ __ __ __ __ __ __ __ __ __ __.

Use the circled letters to form the answer to this jumble. Clue: What is one type of injury that has a high risk of infection because the injury is not exposed to air?

__ __ __ __ __ __ __ __

Identifying Pressure Points

Use Figure 32-8 of the textbook to label the pressure points in Figure 32-1.

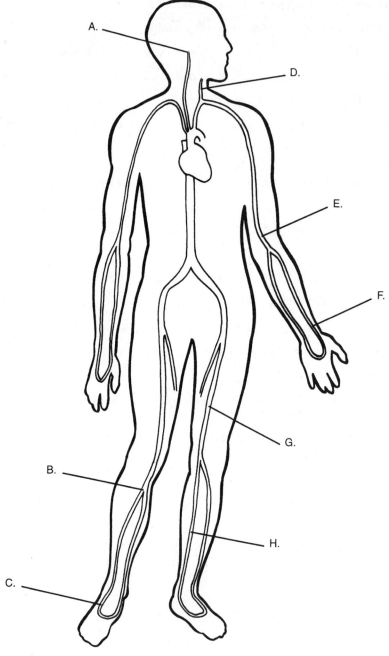

Figure 32-1

A. _____

B. _____

C. _____

D. _____

E. _____

F. _____

G. _____

H. _____

Inventing First Aid Reminders

Acronyms, or sayings made by letters, are often used to assist the memory. "ABCs" is an acronym commonly used in first aid to list the steps of assessment and the cardiopulmonary resuscitation (CPR) procedure. Choose one of the first aid situations from the textbook and design an acronym to help you remember the steps of care.

LETTER		ACTION STEP
_____	=	_____
_____	=	_____
_____	=	_____
_____	=	_____
_____	=	_____
_____	=	_____
_____	=	_____
_____	=	_____
_____	=	_____
_____	=	_____

Applying Your Knowledge

1. In 2010, the American Heart Association announced new CPR guidelines. Explain why the new acronym for bystander CPR is now "CAB" instead of "ABC"?

_____

_____

_____

2. Give one other acronym you have used to remember an action plan.

_____

_____

_____

Emergency Health Careers

Emergency Health Skills and Qualities

List three personal qualities and skills that are important in emergency careers.

1. _____

2. _____

3. _____

Identifying Emergency Health Careers

Use the textbook to provide the missing information about emergency careers in Table 32-1.

TABLE 32-1 Emergency Health Careers

CAREER TITLE	YEARS OF EDUCATION	DESCRIPTION OF JOB DUTIES AND OPPORTUNITIES	CREDENTIALS REQUIRED
			EMT-I; certification required
		Works in prehospital situation to provide care to victim of accident, injury, or illness; may administer medications and monitor ECG equipment	EMT-P; certification required
			BSN, licensure required
	110 or more hours of supervised education		
			AA and ARC offer classes for education

INVESTIGATIONS

Casualty Simulation

Read all of the directions before beginning this activity. Laboratory activities should be completed under the supervision of a qualified professional only.

Equipment and Supplies

Newspaper
Pillows
Sheets

Directions

1. Choose a partner to role play one of the casualty simulations.
2. Choose a third person to act as the victim.
3. Consult with your partner for 3 minutes about the situation before beginning the role play.
4. Other members of the class may act as observers and evaluate the care given to the victim, using Figure 32-2.
5. Switch roles to complete the simulations.

```
┌─────────────────────────────────────────────────────────────────┐
│            EVALUATION SCALE FOR CASUALTY SIMULATION               │
│                                                                   │
│   Communicates effectively with victim          ____/ 10 points   │
│   Communicates effectively with partner         ____/ 5 points    │
│   Volunteers pertinent information about assessment               │
│      and first aid treatment                    ____/ 5 points    │
│   Assesses victim for known and unknown injuries ____/ 10 points  │
│   Correctly treats injuries                     ____/ 10 points   │
│   Gives first aid care quickly                  ____/ 5 points    │
│   Uses safety measures to protect victim and selves ____/ 5 points│
│   TOTAL TEAM SCORE:                             ____/ 50 points   │
└─────────────────────────────────────────────────────────────────┘
```

Figure 32-2

Casualty Simulation Victims

Situation One

Your victim was working on a power pole and touched a live wire while unsuccessfully trying to break a fall. The fall was approximately 20 feet. His right hand has a third-degree burn diagonally across the palm from contact with the wire. He also has some first- and second-degree burns around the area of the third-degree burn. The victim is responsive and complaining of severe pain in his lower right arm.

Situation Two

Your victim was kicked in the chest by a horse. You find her sitting against a fence post. She is dazed and confused but responsive. She is complaining of numbness and a tingling sensation in her left arm. You can see that the left arm is displaced in a downward direction from a break in the left clavicle.

Situation Three

Your victim was running up the bleachers at school and slipped. He fell down the bleachers to the concrete below. He has a compound fracture of the left femur with moderate bleeding. He is responsive and complains of difficulty breathing.

Situation Four

Your victim is a student in a chemistry class. He knocked over a gas burner and some flammable liquid chemicals. The burning liquid ignited his shirt and jeans. The teacher pushed the student under the shower and put out the fire with water. The victim has first- and second-degree burns on his chest and both upper legs. He is pacing around the room and screaming that the pain is unbearable.

Situation Five

Your victim was injured in a car accident. She has a fractured jaw and a closed fracture of the right lower arm. She is responsive but confused.

Situation Six

Your victim had an accident while riding an all-terrain vehicle in the desert. You do not know how long he was in the desert after the accident. His breathing is rapid and shallow. His pulse is very fast. He is not responsive. His skin is hot and dry to the touch. A bruise is visible on his left upper arm, and the bone looks out of place in that area.

Drawing Conclusions

1. What first aid consideration must be made for all of the victims?

_____

_____

_____

2. For each of the emergency situations described, list one measure that might have been used to prevent the injury.

Situation 1: _____

_____

_____

Situation 2: _____

_____

_____

Situation 3: _____

_____

_____

Situation 4: _____

_____

_____

Situation 5: _____

_____

_____

Situation 6: _____

_____

_____

CRITICAL THINKING

Understanding Survival

The newspaper headlines read, "Dead Tot Improving at Hospital." The article reported the story of a boy age 2 years who, wearing only pajamas, wandered from his home in subzero temperatures. He was found frozen in the snow hours later with a core body temperature of 60° F. He had no vital signs present, and all of his extremities were frozen. Health care workers resuscitated the boy and slowly returned his body temperature to normal. Although he had some damaged tissue from the freezing, the boy suffered no heart or brain damage from the ordeal.

A Chicago boy fell through the ice while sledding by Lake Michigan and was submerged for about 20 minutes. Doctors were able to bring the boy back to life by maintaining life support and placing him in a drug-induced coma while raising his body temperature to normal.

Examining the Evidence

1. What may have allowed these boys to live through "death" without apparent brain damage due to lack of oxygen?

_____

_____

_____

2. What other injuries might occur as a result of the body tissues freezing?

_____

_____

_____

3. How did the drug-induced coma help the Chicago boy in his recovery?

_____

_____

_____

"RICE" Is Nice

Athletic trainers work to provide sports enthusiasts with a safe and productive training schedule. They are also the primary emergency caregivers when an athlete is injured during practice or an athletic event. An acronym used by trainers to give immediate care for minor injuries to muscles, tendons, and ligaments is "RICE" or "ICE-R." After the initial assessment to rule out fractures, the athletic trainer wants to control bleeding, inflammation, muscle spasm, and pain resulting from the injury. RICE stands for rest, ice, compression, and elevation.

With RICE treatment, the activity is stopped if pain is severe. Ice is placed on the injured area for 15 to 20 minutes. An elastic wrap is placed around the area affected. The painful area is elevated above the heart when possible.

Examining the Evidence

1. Why is the "ice" part of RICE used for muscular injuries?

_____

_____

_____

2. Why is the "compression" part of RICE used for muscular injuries?

_____

_____

_____

3. Why is the "elevation" part of RICE used for muscular injuries?

_____

_____

_____

4. Why is the "rest" part of RICE used for muscular injuries?

_____

_____

_____

5. In addition to preventing further injury, what is one other goal the athletic trainer would have in the treatment of a muscular injury?

_____

_____

_____

INTERNET ACTIVITIES

Education and Career Research

Use the following links, other Internet resources, and information available by telephone or mail inquiry to determine the educational cost of one emergency health career and the salary that might be earned in the local area. Use the information to complete Table 32-2.

Suggested Websites

Salary.com: http://salary.com
Monster.com: http://monster.com
Occupational Outlook Handbook: http://www.bls.gov/oco/
American Heart Association (AHA): http://www.americaheart.org
National Association of Emergency Medical Technicians (NAEMT): http://www.naemt.org/

TABLE 32-2 Education and Career Research

CAREER	INSTITUTION FOR EDUCATION	COST OF EDUCATION	POTENTIAL EARNINGS

33 Information and Administration Careers

VAPID VOCABULARY

Complete the crossword puzzle below using the Key Terms.

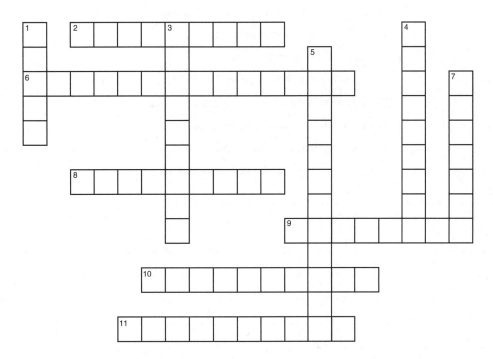

ACROSS

2 Lacking some important part
6 Management, performance of executive responsibilities and duties
8 Speaking words to be written by another person; may be recorded
9 An individual occurrence or event occurring in connection with something else; a reportable variance
10 To make a written copy of dictated or recorded matter
11 Fee that considers both the usual fee charged by a practitioner for a particular service and the fee charged by other practitioners for the same service

DOWN

1 Collection of written materials relating to the health care of a patient
3 Fee charged by similar practitioners for a service in the same economic and geographical area
4 Payment by contract by one party to another in which the second party guarantees the first party against financial loss from a specific event
5 Private and secret; may be protected by law
7 Financial help in time of illness, retirement, or unemployment

ABBREVIATIONS

Match each of the following abbreviations with the phrase that best describes it's meaning or function. Then write the phrase of name for each of the abbreviations in the spaces below.

Abbreviation	Meaning or Function
1. _____ AHIMA	a. Certification for medical staff services personnel
2. _____ CEBS	b. Certified healthcare worker who checks credentials
3. _____ CPCS	c. Health information professional association
4. _____ FCRA	d. List of plans to ensure patient safety
5. _____ HIM	e. Manager of health information
6. _____ JCAHO	f. Organization that defines guidelines for background checks
7. _____ NAMSS	g. Organization that oversees healthcare facilities
8. _____ NPSG	h. Professional organization for medical staff services
9. _____ RHIT	i. Registered manager of health information
10. _____ RRA	j. Registered technician of health information

1. AHIMA: _____

2. CEBS: _____

3. CPCS: _____

4. FCRA: _____

5. HIM: _____

6. JCAHO: _____

7. NAMSS: _____

8. NPSG: _____

9. RHIT: _____

10. RRA: _____

JUST THE FACTS

1. Careers in _ _ _ _ _ _ _ _ _ _ _ _ _ _ _ _ _ include health care facility managers, supervisors, medical secretaries, unit coordinators, and medical records personnel.

2. Administrators _ _ _ _ _ _ _ _ _ _ services, hiring, and training of personnel.

3. Patient representatives, or _ _ _ _ _ _ _ _ _ _, help patients to understand the health care policies and procedures of the facility, obtain services, and make informed decisions about their care.

4. The _ _ _ _ _ _ _ _ _ _ _ _ _ _ _ _ _ is employed by institutions and private facilities, such as a doctor's office, to assist in administration of services.

5. The health unit coordinator (HUC) performs _ _ _ _ _ _ _ _ _ _ _ activities for the nursing unit.

6. Medical _ _ _ _ _ _ _ personnel organize, analyze, and generate data relating to patient records.

7. The medical _ listens to and types information

   to provide a permanent record from a variety of audio equipment.

8. ◯ _ _ _ _ _ _   _ _ _ _ _ _ _ _   _ _ _ _ _ _ _ _ _ _ _ provide

   access to information by practicing professionals, researchers, and students.

9. Orderliness of equipment and supplies used in the work area provides a secure environment for maintaining the

   _ _ _ _ _ _ _ _ _ _ _ _ _ _ _ _ _ of patient records.

10. ◯ _ _ _ _ _ _ must be accurate, legible, complete, and organized to provide efficient care.

   Use the circled letters to form the answer to this jumble. Clue: What is the collection of papers, test results, and patient information called?

   _ _ _ _ _

CONCEPT APPLICATIONS

Composing a Business Letter

On your own sheet of paper, type or print a letter using the following information. You work for a medical doctor as a front office assistant. You have noticed that the account of Mrs. Adrienne Jones is overdue. Insurance has paid for all of the expenses of her care except for a $180 visit for a second opinion with an associate in the office. Your doctor asks you to write a letter to Mrs. Jones to remind her of the fee due. The doctor asks you to keep in mind as you are writing the letter that Mrs. Jones's husband of 50 years died 6 months ago and that she might not be familiar with billing and insurance procedures. Mrs. Jones's address is 2325 S. Wilshire Blvd., Any town, USA, 00345. You may create your own doctor's name and address.

Applying Your Knowledge

1. Explain why you think you should or should not mention the loss of Mrs. Jones's husband in the letter.

   _____
   _____
   _____

2. Design a standard form letter to indicate fees that are due so that only the name, address, service performed, and amount owed need to be added before mailing.

   _____
   _____
   _____

Keeping a Budget Ledger

Use the daily log of charges and receipts in Figure 33-1 to answer the questions and complete the receipt form in Figure 33-2 for client Dwight Nelson.

Applying Your Knowledge

1. What is the total of the payments for the day?

   _____

2. Which clients do not owe any money to date?

   _____

3. What is the total for checks received on the date shown?

   _____

Chapter **33** **Information and Administration Careers**

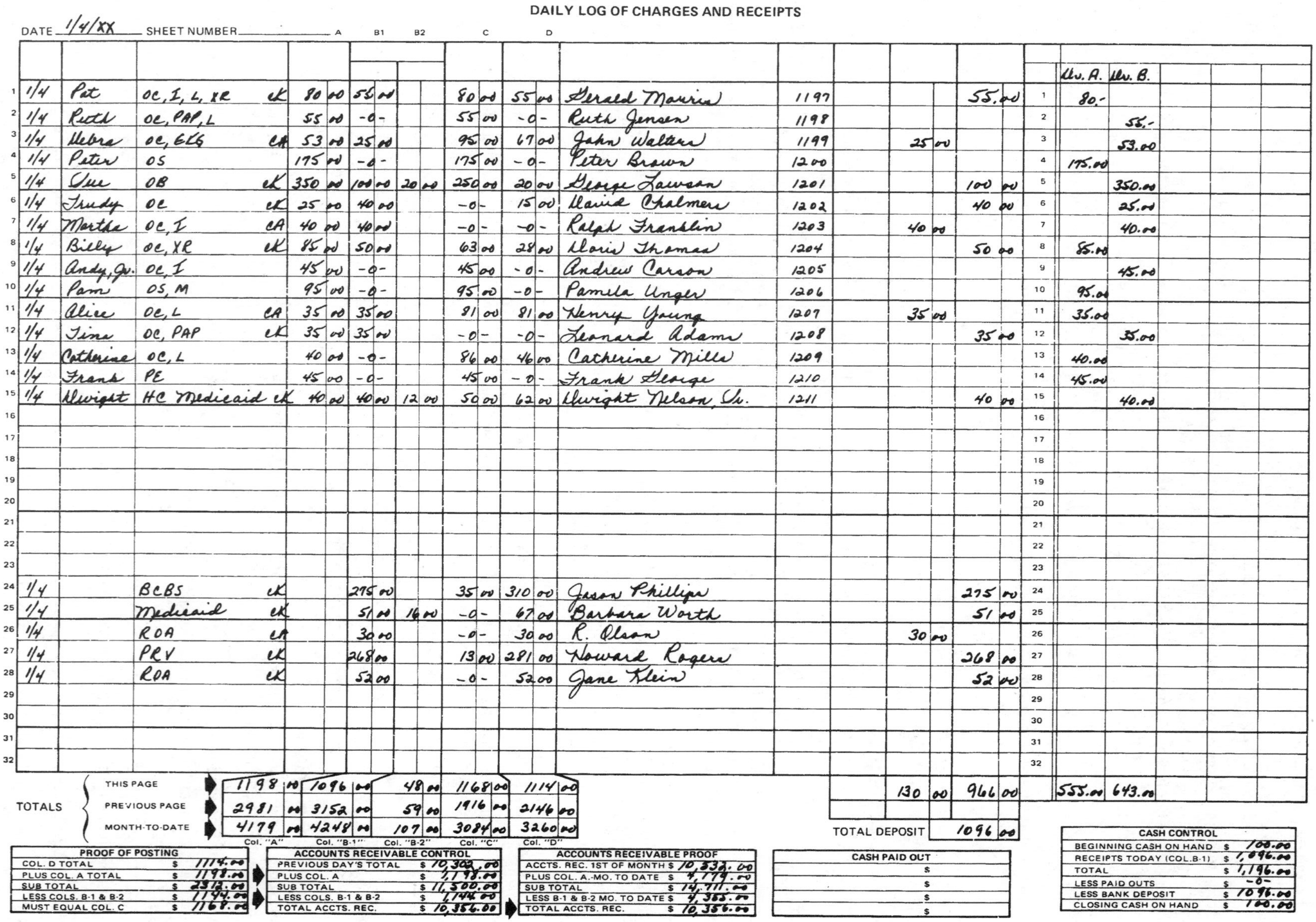

DAILY LOG OF CHARGES AND RECEIPTS

DATE 1/4/XX SHEET NUMBER

					A	B1	B2	C	D							Dr. A.	Dr. B.
1	1/4	Pat	OC, I, L, XR	ck	80 00	55 00		80 00	55 00	Gerald Morris	1197			55.00	1	80.-	
2	1/4	Ruth	OC, PAP, L		55 00	-0-		55 00	-0-	Ruth Jensen	1198				2		55.-
3	1/4	Debra	OC, EKG	CA	53 00	25 00		95 00	67 00	John Walters	1199		25 00		3		53.00
4	1/4	Peter	OS		175 00	-0-		175 00	-0-	Peter Brown	1200				4	175.00	
5	1/4	Sue	OB	ck	350 00	100 00	20 00	250 00	20 00	George Lawson	1201			100 00	5		350.00
6	1/4	Trudy	OC	ck	25 00	40 00		-0-	15 00	David Chalmers	1202			40 00	6		25.00
7	1/4	Martha	OC, I	CA	40 00	40 00		-0-	-0-	Ralph Franklin	1203		40 00		7		40.00
8	1/4	Billy	OC, XR	ck	85 00	50 00		63 00	28 00	Doris Thomas	1204			50 00	8	85.00	
9	1/4	Andy, Jr.	OC, I		45 00	-0-		45 00	-0-	Andrew Carson	1205				9		45.00
10	1/4	Pam	OS, M		95 00	-0-		95 00	-0-	Pamela Unger	1206				10	95.00	
11	1/4	Alice	OC, L	CA	35 00	35 00		81 00	81 00	Henry Young	1207		35 00		11	35.00	
12	1/4	Tina	OC, PAP	ck	35 00	35 00		-0-	-0-	Leonard Adams	1208			35 00	12		35.00
13	1/4	Catherine	OC, L		40 00	-0-		86 00	46 00	Catherine Mills	1209				13	40.00	
14	1/4	Frank	PE		45 00	-0-		45 00	-0-	Frank George	1210				14	45.00	
15	1/4	Dwight	HC Medicaid	ck	40 00	40 00	12 00	50 00	62 00	Dwight Nelson, Jr.	1211			40 00	15		40.00
16															16		
17															17		
18															18		
19															19		
20															20		
21															21		
22															22		
23															23		
24	1/4		BCBS	ck		275 00		35 00	310 00	Jason Phillips				275 00	24		
25	1/4		Medicaid	ck		51 00	16 00	-0-	67 00	Barbara Worth				51 00	25		
26	1/4		ROA	CA		30 00		-0-	30 00	R. Olson			30 00		26		
27	1/4		PRV	ck		268 00		13 00	281 00	Howard Rogers				268 00	27		
28	1/4		ROA	ck		52 00		-0-	52 00	Jane Klein				52 00	28		
29															29		
30															30		
31															31		
32															32		

TOTALS	Col. "A"	Col. "B-1"	Col. "B-2"	Col. "C"	Col. "D"
THIS PAGE	1198 00	1096 00	48 00	1168 00	1114 00
PREVIOUS PAGE	2981 00	3152 00	59 00	1916 00	2146 00
MONTH-TO-DATE	4179 00	4248 00	107 00	3084 00	3260 00

130 00	966 00		555.00	643.00

TOTAL DEPOSIT 1096 00

PROOF OF POSTING	
COL. D TOTAL	$ 1114.00
PLUS COL. A TOTAL	$ 1198.00
SUB TOTAL	$ 2312.00
LESS COLS. B-1 & B-2	$ 1144.00
MUST EQUAL COL. C	$ 1168.00

ACCOUNTS RECEIVABLE CONTROL	
PREVIOUS DAY'S TOTAL	$ 10,302.00
PLUS COL. A	$ 1,198.00
SUB TOTAL	$ 11,500.00
LESS COLS. B-1 & B-2	$ 1,144.00
TOTAL ACCTS. REC.	$ 10,356.00

ACCOUNTS RECEIVABLE PROOF	
ACCTS. REC. 1ST OF MONTH	$ 10,532.00
PLUS COL. A-MO. TO DATE	$ 4,179.00
SUB TOTAL	$ 14,711.00
LESS B-1 & B-2 MO. TO DATE	$ 4,355.00
TOTAL ACCTS. REC.	$ 10,356.00

CASH PAID OUT	
	$
	$
	$
	$

CASH CONTROL	
BEGINNING CASH ON HAND	$ 100.00
RECEIPTS TODAY (COL. B-1)	$ 1,096.00
TOTAL	$ 1,196.00
LESS PAID OUTS	$ -0-
LESS BANK DEPOSIT	$ 1096.00
CLOSING CASH ON HAND	$ 100.00

Figure 33-1 Daily ledger. (From Cooper M, Cooper D, Burrows N: *The medical assistant*, ed 6, St. Louis, 1993, Mosby.)

Clifford Temperson, MD
1023 Gentileer Drive, Suite 413
Anywhereville, Anystate, 12345

Date ____________ 20 ___ No. 23100

RECEIPT

Received from ____ $ ________

____ Dollars

For ____

Account	________
Payment	________
Balance due	________

___ Cash
___ Check
___ Money order

Received by

____

Figure 33-2 Receipt

Information and Administration Careers

Information and Administration Skills and Qualities

List three personal qualities and skills that are important in information and administration careers.

1. ______________________________
2. ______________________________
3. ______________________________

Identifying Information and Administration Careers

Use the textbook to provide the missing information about information and administration careers in Table 33-1.

TABLE 33-1 Information and Administration Careers

CAREER TITLE	YEARS OF EDUCATION	DESCRIPTION OF JOB DUTIES AND OPPORTUNITIES	CREDENTIALS REQUIRED
			RRA
			CEO
		Duties of receptionist, accountant, and assistant; use telephone	
		Assists the patient to understand health care practices and policies	
			HUC

Applying Your Knowledge

1. A patient might seek help with preparing a living will or resolving a conflict in the facility from the health care worker called a(n) _____.

2. The health care worker who listens to and prints audio recordings of information is called a(n) _____.

3. Access to printed information by health care professionals is often the responsibility of the _____.

4. Individuals who take photographs are often prepared with a _____ education.

5. Analyzing information relating to current trends in the health of a community is probably the responsibility of the _____.

Admitting a Patient

Directions

1. Choose partners to role play the admission of a patient to the facility. Use the admission checklist shown in Figure 33-3.
2. Provide feedback to the person who is doing the admission about the clarity of instruction and his/her manner.
3. Switch roles and perform the admission procedure again.

Drawing Conclusions

1. What types of activities that occur in a hospital might require explanation to a client who has never before been in a hospital?

_____

_____

_____

Date: _____ Time: _____ Introduced: Self _____ Roommate _____

Admitted per: Wheelchair _____ Cart _____ Ambulatory _____ Carried by _____

Age: _____ Sex: M _____ F _____

Condition on admission:

Ambulatory ☐	Feeds self ☐	Admitted by ambulance ☐	Alert ☐
Semiambulatory ☐	Requires help with feeding ☐	From hospital ☐	Forgetful ☐
Chairridden ☐	Continent ☐	From home ☐	Confused ☐
Bedridden ☐	Incontinent ☐	From nursing home ☐	

State of consciousness: Alert _____ Confused _____ Semiconscious _____ Unconscious _____

Emotional state: Calm _____ Nervous _____ Fearful _____ Angry _____ Depressed _____

Pain: No _____ Yes _____ Where _____

Vital signs: BP _____ T _____ P _____ R _____ Ht _____ Wt _____

Glasses: Yes _____ No _____ Contact lenses: Yes _____ No _____ Hearing aid: Yes _____ No _____

Dentures: Yes _____ No _____ Artificial limb: Yes _____ No _____

Artificial eye: Yes _____ No _____ Right _____ Left _____ Pacemaker: Yes _____ No _____

Orientation to environment:

Call light _____ Emergency light _____ Bed controls _____ Bedside stand _____ Closet _____

Drawers _____ Bathroom _____ Mealtime _____ Visiting hours _____

Information obtained from: Patient _____ Spouse _____ Parent: M _____ F _____ Other _____

Other observations and comments: _____

_____

Show all body marks: scars, bruises, cuts, decubiti, ulcers, and discolorations (birth marks should not be shown).

Signed _____

Figure 33-3 Admission checklist.

365

2. Why is it important to note all scars, bruises, decubitus ulcers, and other body marks on admission?

_____

_____

_____

CRITICAL THINKING

Verifying Medical Records

One of the responsibilities of medical records personnel is to verify or check the medical record. For example, the pages of the chart should be correctly labeled with the patient's name.

List three other items that would need to be verified to ensure the accuracy of the chart.

1. _____

2. _____

3. _____

Personnel Issues

Place yourself in the role of a manager in a health care facility. It is time for the first 3-month employee review in the following two situations. Prepare a written evaluation of at least two paragraphs for each of the two individuals described. You may create additional facts as desired for your evaluation. These situations may also be used for role playing.

Situation One

Overall, the performance of Nancy Be Good is adequate for this level of job entry. However, some problems have been noted by you and mentioned by her fellow workers. Nancy is late for work one or two times a week, always by just a few minutes. Additionally, she takes a few extra minutes for break several times each week, again usually less than 5 minutes. She does not show initiative in finding tasks to be performed when she finishes her assigned work. Also, she uses slang terms instead of correct medical terminology when talking with staff members, doctors, and patients.

Examining the Evidence

1. Which issue about Nancy's behavior do you consider the most important to improve? Explain why.

_____

_____

_____

2. Why is arriving late to work or returning late from break a problem even when it is only a few minutes?

_____

_____

_____

3. What would be an appropriate method and time period for following up on this employee review?

_____

_____

_____

Situation Two

John Longface is having some personal problems at home. His work has been above average in the past but is now being performed inadequately. The problem started about 2 weeks before this review. His performance is too poor for you to allow it to continue. The most recent incident was his absence from work without notifying anyone that he would be gone. When you called his residence to see if he had left for work, his wife informed you that he was in bed and did not plan to come in.

Examining the Evidence

1. Explain why it is unacceptable to let personal problems affect work performance.

   _____
   _____
   _____

2. How do people "rise above" or "put aside" personal problems when at work?

   _____
   _____
   _____

3. What would be an appropriate method and time period for following up on this employee review?

   _____
   _____
   _____

INTERNET ACTIVITIES

Education and Career Research

Use the following links, other Internet resources, and information available by telephone or mail inquiry to determine the educational cost of one information and administration career and the salary that might be earned in the local area. Use the information to complete Table 33-2.

Suggested Websites

Salary.com: http://salary.com
Monster.com: http://monster.com
Occupational Outlook Handbook: http://www.bls.gov/oco/
Joint Commission Quality Check®: http://www.qualitycheck.org/consumer/searchQCR.aspx
National Association Medical Staff Services (NAMSS): http://www.namss.org/
American Health Information Management Association (AHIMA): http://www.ahima.org

TABLE 33-2 Education and Career Research

CAREER	INSTITUTION FOR EDUCATION	COST OF EDUCATION	POTENTIAL EARNINGS

VAPID VOCABULARY

Complete the crossword puzzle using the Key Terms.

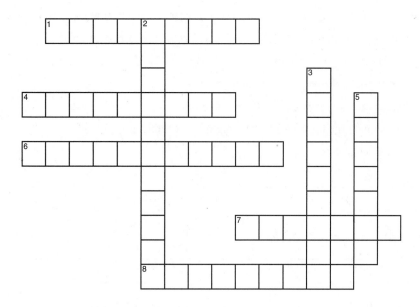

ACROSS

1 Part of the universe, including the air (atmosphere), earth (lithosphere), and water (hydrosphere), in which living organisms exist
4 Condition of being defiled or impure
6 Organic compound made of hydrogen and carbon only
7 Unit used to express ratio of power between two sounds
8 Living organisms and nonliving elements interacting in a specific area

DOWN

2 Composed of separate particles or pieces
3 Poison used to destroy pests of any kind
5 Physical or chemical agent that induces genetic mutation or change

ABBREVIATIONS

Match each of the following abbreviations with the phrase that best describes its meaning or function. Then write the phrase or name for each of the abbreviations in the spaces provided.

Abbreviation	Meaning or Function
1. _____ AST	a. Certified health care worker who services and maintains biomedical equipment
2. _____ CBET	b. Certified health care worker who services and maintains laboratory equipment
3. _____ CDC	c. Certified health care worker who services and maintains radiologic equipment
4. _____ CLES	d. Federal organization that reports statistics regarding environmental hazard exposure
5. _____ CRES	e. Health care worker who collects and analyzes air and water samples
6. _____ dB	f. Low-frequency energy emissions
7. _____ EHT	g. Measurement of loudness or volume
8. _____ EMF	h. Organization that certifies radiation monitors
9. _____ NRRPT	i. Professional organization for operating room technicians
10. _____ ORT	j. Surgical technician

1. AST: _____

2. CBET: _____

3. CDC: _____

4. CLES: _____

5. CRES: _____

6. dB: _____

7. EHT: _____

8. EMF: _____

9. NRRPT: _____

10. ORT: _____

JUST THE FACTS

1. Most _ _ _ _ _ _ _ _ _ workers are not seen by the person receiving the service.

2. _ _ Ⓞ _ _ _ _ _ _ supervise food operations to meet the patients' needs and provide counseling on nutrition.

3. The type of _ _ Ⓞ _ _ _ _ _ is determined by the physician's order and special needs of the patient.

4. The _ Ⓞ _ _ _ _ _ _ _ _ _ _ _ Ⓞ _ _ engineer analyzes contamination problems to establish methods and equipment to prevent pollution.

5. _ _ _ _ _ _ _ Ⓞ _ _ _ _ _ _ identify existing and potential hazards in conditions and practices.

6. _ _ _ _ _ Ⓞ _ _ _ analyze and regulate the quality of the environment as it is affected by living organisms.

7. _ _ _ _ _ _ _ _ _ services include groundskeeping, housekeeping, and other personnel needed to run a large institution.

8. The Ⓞ _ _ _ _ _ _ _ _   _ _ _ Ⓞ _ _ _ _ _ _ _, or operating room technologist, maintains the sterile field during surgery and passes instruments to the surgeon.

9. _ _ _ _ _ _ Ⓞ Ⓞ _ _ _ _ _ _ _, or sterile supply technicians, sterilize, assemble, clean, and store diagnostic and surgical equipment.

10. The _ Ⓞ _ _ _ _ _ _ _ is the air, crust of the earth, and water.

Use the circled letters to form the answer to this jumble. Clue: What do more than 23 million Americans have in common?

_ _ _ _ _ _ _ _   _ _ _ _

CONCEPT APPLICATIONS

Identifying the Parts and Functions of the Chain of Life

Use Figure 34-6 of the textbook to label the diagram of the chain of life in Figure 34-1. In the spaces provided in Table 34-1, explain the role played by each of the parts of the chain in recycling of the biosphere's resources.

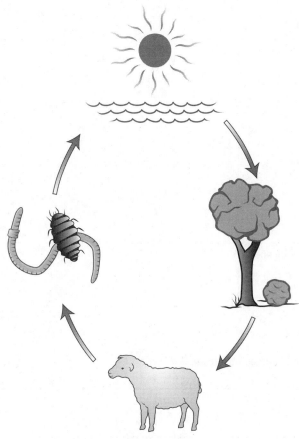

Figure 34-1

TABLE 34-1 Functions of the Chain of Life

PART OF THE CHAIN	ROLE IN THE BIOSPHERE
1. Sunlight, water, air, organic compounds, and nutrients	
2. Plants on land and water	
3. Herbivores and carnivores	
4. Decomposers	

Using the Epidemiological Approach

Use the epidemiological approach provided in the textbook to identify and solve the health problem described.

Problem Description

Your club participated in the school picnic. To raise funds, you sold soft drinks. Other clubs provided hamburgers, pizza, several types of salad, cookies, and ice cream.

Approximately 2 hours after the picnic, 40 students became very ill and had to be taken to a local health care facility.

The administration decided that no more food-related activities would be allowed on the school campus. Your club would like the administration to reconsider.

You plan to investigate this problem. You may invent information resulting from your investigation needed to solve the problem. Complete the following chart to show the solution you found through your imaginary investigation.

EPIDEMIOLOGICAL METHOD		
Step 1:	Identify the problem.	
Step 2:	Identify the illness.	
Step 3:	Identify the source of the problem.	
Step 4:	Prevent further incidence.	

Applying Your Knowledge

1. What are three food-related sources of intestinal disorders?

_____

_____

_____

2. How could the epidemiological approach be used to trace the source of an outbreak of hepatitis A to a restaurant worker who carries the virus?

_____

_____

_____

3. For what other health-related problems could the epidemiological approach be used?

_____

_____

_____

Designing a Health Care Environment

Use the information you have learned from the chapter to design a health care environment that includes therapeutic and functional aspects, such as color, decor, and furnishings. It should also provide organizational spaces to prevent clutter and promote safety considerations. You may design a hospital room, a hospital unit (floor), a surgical or examination suite, or a facility of your choice. Your teacher may ask you to provide your design as a written description, a poster, or a three-dimensional model.

Environmental Careers

Environmental Health Skills and Qualities

List three personal qualities and skills that are important in environmental health careers.

1. _____

2. _____

3. _____

Identifying Environmental Health Careers

Use the textbook to provide the missing information about environmental health careers in Table 34-2.

TABLE 34-2 Environmental Careers

CAREER TITLE	YEARS OF EDUCATION	DESCRIPTION OF JOB DUTIES AND OPPORTUNITIES	CREDENTIALS REQUIRED
		Modify facilities for environmental protection, recommend equipment to meet government standards	
		Analyze and regulate the quality of the environment, pollution analysis	
			MS or PhD preferred; registration available
		Counsel patient in methods to reduce weight	
		Provide equipment and supplies in facilities	

Applying Your Knowledge

1. Health care workers who provide services that are not generally seen by the public are called

   _____.

2. A 2-year associate degree is needed for the health care worker who plans menus and supervises the production of

   food and is called a _____.

3. Analysis of contamination problems and determination of how they occurred are performed by the

   _____.

4. Health physics technicians are also called _____.

5. Certification as a specialist in public health may be granted for health care workers called

   _____.

Water Analysis

Read all of the directions before beginning this activity. Laboratory activities should be completed under the supervision of a qualified professional only.

Equipment and Supplies

Incubator
Inoculating loop
Litmus paper
Microscope
Secchi disk
Sterile agar plate
Thermometer
Water samples collected in sterile containers

Directions

1. Collect a water sample in a sterile container. Elements of the water that may indicate pollution include the presence of animal and plant life. The specimen must be collected in a sterile container to prevent contamination from other sources.
2. Observe and record the temperature of the water. Water temperature varies with the climate, oxygen content, and depth of the water sample.
3. Observe and record the turbidity of the water. The turbidity, or clarity, of the water can be determined by the amount of light that passes through it or by use of a Secchi disk. Water with high turbidity may be unacceptable for use by humans.
4. Observe and record the odor of the water. Odor may result from chemicals, organisms, or organic materials in the water. Odor does not necessarily indicate pollution of the water, but it is undesirable.
5. Using a microscope, observe the water and record the presence of life forms in the sample. The animals and plants that live in a body of water are indicators of its oxygen and other content. Microscopic life forms may indicate that the water is unacceptable for use by humans.
6. Observe and record the uses of the water sample area. Water may be used for recreational or industrial purposes. Litter in the water may indicate pollution from inappropriate use.
7. Measure and record the pH of the water sample. Litmus paper can be used to indicate the concentration of acid or alkaline materials in the water sample. The acidity of the water determines whether algae will grow and the relative quantity of minerals, or hardness, of the water.
8. Prepare and incubate a streak culture plate to determine the presence of microscopic bacteria in the sample. Record the results in Table 34-3.
9. Determine the acceptability of the water sample for its intended use. Drinking water should have a neutral pH, be free of microorganisms, have no odor, and be at an appropriate temperature.

TABLE 34-3   Water Analysis Comparison

TYPE OF WATER SAMPLE	TAP	POND
Date and site of water collection		
Temperature of water at time of collection		
Turbidity		
Odor		
Description of microscopic organisms		
Uses of the water sampled		
pH of water sample		
Description of streak plate growth		

Drawing Conclusions

1. Why is the presence of microscopic organisms in water important in determining whether it may be used for drinking and swimming?

_____

_____

_____

2. Explain whether the water samples you tested are safe for drinking.

_____

_____

_____

3. Which health professional collects and analyzes air and water samples under the supervision of the sanitarian?

_____

4. What are three sources of water contamination?

_____

_____

_____

CRITICAL THINKING

Respiratory Effects of Chemical Exposure

The functional units of the respiratory system are directly exposed to the environment. The surface of the lungs provides the largest exposed area of the body. The surface area of the lungs is 70 to $100\,m^2$; by comparison, the surface area of the digestive system is $10\,m^2$ and that of the skin is only $2\,m^2$. Harmful exposure to poisonous substances occurs very quickly through the lung tissue.

Toxins or poisonous substances that can be inhaled are divided into the following categories:

1. Asphyxiates—Gases that deprive the body of oxygen (e.g., carbon dioxide, nitrogen, cyanide, neon, and argon)
2. Irritants—Chemicals that irritate the air passages (e.g., chlorine, hydrochloric acid, and ammonia)
3. Necrosis producers—Gases that result in cell death (e.g., ozone and nitrogen dioxide)
4. Fibrosis producers—Substances that result in the formation of fibrotic tissues (e.g., asbestos and silicates)
5. Allergens—Substances that produce an allergic response (e.g., isocyanates and sulfur dioxide)
6. Carcinogens—Substances that cause the formation of cancerous cells (e.g., cigarette smoke, asbestos, and arsenic)

Examining the Evidence

1. Which of the toxin categories include most of the particulates in air pollution?

_____

_____

_____

2. To which of the toxins listed are you exposed?

_____

_____

_____

3. What are two methods you might use to limit your exposure to the toxins described?

_____

_____

_____

4. Carbon monoxide is known to bind to the hemoglobin molecule 200 times more readily than oxygen. What effect does this have in the body?

_____

_____

_____

5. What are two common sources of carbon monoxide?

_____

_____

_____

Pneumonic Plague

Widespread panic broke out in a city in western India in September, 1994, when an outbreak of pneumonic plague occurred. More than 200,000 people fled the city, trying to avoid a national epidemic. By October the World Health Organization announced that the plague was under control, following the reported deaths of up to 300 people.

Pneumonic plague is caused by the bacterium *Yersinia pestis*. It affects animals such as rodents but can be transmitted to people by fleas. The infection can then be spread from one person to another by airborne droplets.

Examining the Evidence

1. The Centers for Disease Control and Prevention usually imposes a quarantine to prevent the spread of an unknown or infectious agent. Why would this be an important response?

_____

_____

_____

2. How might this plague be contained?

_____

_____

_____

Radiation Testing

In October, 1994, the President's Advisory Committee on Human Radiation Experiments revealed that thousands of secret experiments using radiation had been conducted between 1944 and 1974. Tests included the release of radioactive particles into the environment and their injection into human beings. Approximately 23,000 people were involved in these studies, some without their knowledge. The Departments of Energy and Defense still refuse to release all documents involved in the testing.

Examining the Evidence

1. Most individuals involved in secret tests would not know their risk of complications. Why do or do you not think that these individuals should be informed now?

_____

_____

_____

2. One action under consideration by the advisory committee is financial compensation of victims of testing. Why do or do you not agree with this action?

_____

_____

_____

3. What kinds of safeguards protect the public from secret testing today?

_____

_____

_____

4. Do some research to discover at least one other type of environmental or public health risk caused by the action of the government or some other agency. Record your findings here.

_____

_____

_____

INTERNET ACTIVITIES

Education and Career Research

Use the following links, other Internet resources, and information available by telephone or mail inquiry to determine the educational cost of one environmental career and the salary that might be earned in the local area. Use the information to complete Table 34-4.

Suggested Websites

Salary.com: http://salary.com
Monster.com: http://monster.com
Occupational Outlook Handbook: http://www.bls.gov/oco/
American Dietetic Association: http://www.eatright.org/
Association of Surgical Technologists: http://www.ast.org/

TABLE 34-4 Education and Career Research

CAREER	INSTITUTION FOR EDUCATION	COST OF EDUCATION	POTENTIAL EARNINGS

35 Biotechnology Research and Development Careers

VAPID VOCABULARY

Complete the crossword puzzle using the Key Terms.

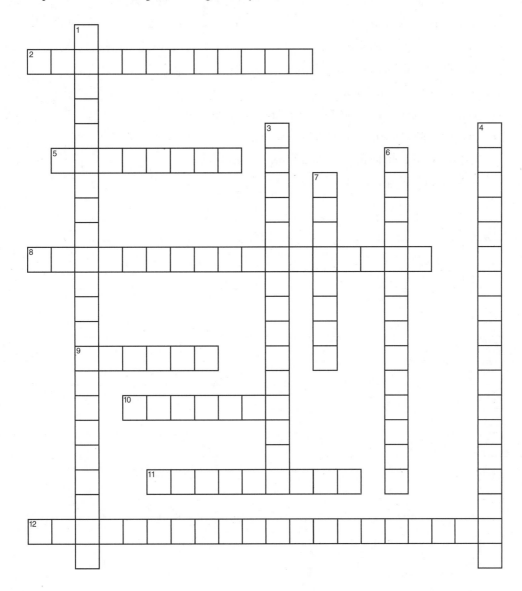

ACROSS

2 Chemical change that is brought about by the action of an enzyme or microorganism
5 A drug, vaccine, or antitoxin that is made from living organisms
8 Choosing the parents of offspring to enhance development of desired traits (two words)
9 Protein that acts as a catalyst in the cell
10 A type of media made of sugar molecules taken from seaweed and used for electrophoresis
11 Pertaining to the courts of law
12 Large nucleic acid molecule that makes up chromosomes (two words)

DOWN

1 Injection of semen into the uterine canal, unrelated to sexual intercourse (two words)
3 Movement of charged suspended particles through a medium in response to an electric field
4 Identical cells or cells originating from the same cell (two words)
6 Collection, classification, and analysis of biological information such as molecular and genetic data
7 Study of the methods for controlling the characteristics of humans

Chapter **35 Biotechnology Research and Development Careers**

ABBREVIATIONS

Match each of the following abbreviations with the phrase that best describes its meaning or function. Then write the phrase or name for each of the abbreviations in the spaces provided.

Abbreviation	Meaning or Function
1. _____ BRCA1	a. Federal organization that approves vaccines
2. _____ DNA	b. Federal organization that provides information on biotechnology
3. _____ FDA	c. Federal organization that regulates genetically modified food
4. _____ HGP	d. Federal organization that sets guidelines for transfer and manipulation of DNA
5. _____ HIV	e. Gene that causes breast cancer
6. _____ mtDNA	f. Identification and sequencing of all human chromosomes
7. _____ NCBI	g. Large nuclear molecule that determines characteristics
8. _____ NIH	h. Molecule that changes DNA information into proteins
9. _____ tRNA	i. Non-nuclear molecule that determines characteristics
10. _____ USDA	j. Virus that causes AIDS

1. BRCA1: _____

2. DNA: _____

3. FDA: _____

4. HGP: _____

5. HIV: _____

6. mtDNA: _____

7. NCBI: _____

8. NIH: _____

9. tRNA: _____

10. USDA: _____

Chapter 35 Biotechnology Research and Development Careers

1. Biotechnology applies scientific and engineering techniques to the manipulation of the _ _ _ O _ of living organisms.

2. Scientists have been using natural techniques of biotechnology such as
_ _ _ _ _ O _ _ _ _ _ _, _ _ _ _ _ _ _ _ _ _ breeding, and
_ _ _ _ _ _ O _ _ _ insemination for many years.

3. _ _ _ O _ _ guidelines for the transfer and manipulation of DNA have been established by the National Institutes of Health.

4. Biotechnologists may work in many fields of practice, including research, _ O _ _ _ _ _ _ _ _,
_ _ _ _ _ _ _ _ _ _ _, and teaching.

5. Medical biotechnologists work with the production of _ _ _ _ _ _ _ _ _ _ Ofor the diagnosis or treatment of disease.

6. _ _ _ _ _ O _ _ _ _ _ study patterns of inheritance and develop methods to influence genetic information.

7. _ _ _ _ _ _ _ _ _ _ _ _ _ _ O _ _ _ _ _ _ _ is a molecule that, by the sequencing of its components, determines all of the characteristics of living things.

8. The O _ _ _ _ _ _ _ _ _ _ _ _ O _ _ _ _ _ is an international effort to identify and sequence all of the human chromosomes.

9. Some genetically modified foods in development include edible _ _ _ _ _ _ _ O, therapeutic
O _ _ _ _ _ _ _ _, and _ _ _ _ _ _ _ _ _ O _ produced by plants.

10. Some of the techniques of biotechnology include gene _ _ O _ _ _ _ and gene
_ _ _ _ _ _ _ _ _, or O _ _ _ _ _ _ _ _ _ _ _ DNA.

Use the circled letters to form the answer to this jumble. Clue: What is the name of the biotechnology technique that may be used to identify suspects in a crime or to determine paternity?

_ _ _ _ _ _ _ _ _ _ _ _ _ _ _ _ _

Chapter **35** **Biotechnology Research and Development Careers**

Identifying the Structure of DNA

Use Figure 35-5 of the textbook to label the diagram of DNA in Figure 35-1.

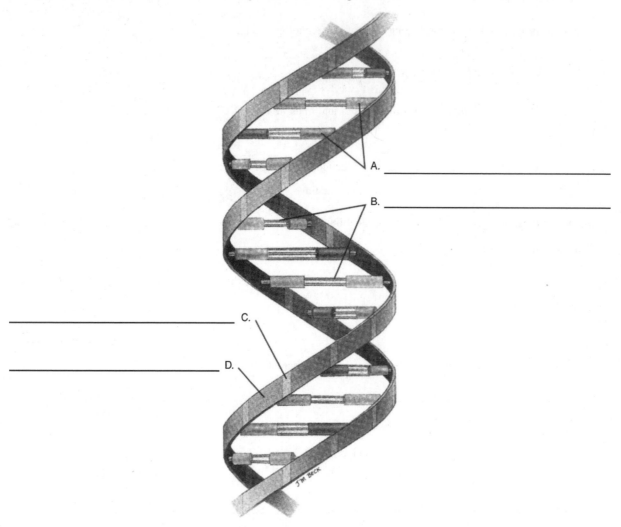

Figure 35-1   Courtesy of Joan M. Beck.

Settling a Paternity Suit

Figure 35-2 is the DNA analysis results from a disputed paternity suit. The mother claims that one of the three men tested is the father of her child. Testing for blood type was inconclusive. The mother has blood type O. The child is blood type O. The three men have blood types A, B, and O.

Mother	Child	Father #1	Father #2	Father #3
───────	───────			
		───────		───────
	───────		───────	───────
───────	───────			
───────		───────		
	───────		───────	
	───────	───────	───────	
───────	───────			───────
───────		───────		
	───────		───────	
	───────	───────		───────
───────		───────	───────	
───────	───────			───────

Figure 35-2   DNA Electrophoresis Digest.

Applying Your Knowledge

1. Why would the tests for blood type be inconclusive?

_____

_____

_____

2. Which individual(s) may be eliminated as the potential father of the child?

_____

_____

_____

3. Which individual(s) may not be eliminated as the father of the child?

_____

_____

_____

Chapter **35 Biotechnology Research and Development Careers**

Biotechnology Careers

Biotechnology Skills and Qualities

List three personal qualities and skills that are important in biotechnology careers.

1. _____

2. _____

3. _____

Identifying Biotechnology Careers

Use the textbook to provide the missing information about biotechnology careers in Table 35-1.

TABLE 35-1 Biotechnology Careers

CAREER TITLE	YEARS OF EDUCATION	DESCRIPTION OF JOB DUTIES AND OPPORTUNITIES	CREDENTIALS REQUIRED
		Bioinstrumentation, biothermodynamics, biotransport, biomechanics	
		Conduct research in cell genetics, may work in research, medicine, or forensics	
	Apprenticeship		

Applying Your Knowledge

1. Health care workers who design new devices such as robotic surgical instruments are called _____

2. Information regarding the genetic makeup of an individual may be determined by the _____

3. A 4-year degree in biotechnology qualifies an individual for work as a(n) _____

INVESTIGATIONS

Performing a DNA Extraction

Read all of the directions before beginning this activity. Laboratory activities should be completed under the supervision of a qualified professional only.

Equipment and Supplies

Alcohol
250-mL beaker
Dishwashing liquid
Eyedropper
Glass rod
Hot water bath
Nonpathogenic bacteria (yeast may be used)
Nutrient broth (water for yeast)
Test tube
Test tube holder
Thermometer

Directions

1. Maintain medical asepsis by practicing good handwashing technique.
2. Prepare a broth of nonpathogenic bacteria or mix yeast in water at 50° C to 60° C.
3. Pour approximately 10 mL of bacterial broth into a clean test tube.
4. Add approximately 5 mL of dishwashing liquid to the test tube.
5. Place the test tube in a hot water bath for 15 minutes. Do not exceed 60° C.
6. Use an eyedropper to add alcohol to cover the top of the solution.
7. Gently stir a glass rod into the solution, through the alcohol.
8. Continue to stir the glass rod through the alcohol into the solution.
9. Record your observations.
10. Clean materials as directed by your instructor, and place them in the designated location.

Drawing Conclusions

1. What are the fibers called that collect around the glass tube?

_____

_____

_____

2. Why must the glass rod be turned gently in the solution?

_____

_____

_____

3. What is the purpose of each of the reagents used in the extraction?

_____

_____

_____

CRITICAL THINKING

Genetic Testing

Many genetic tests can now be performed using a simple blood test. Some examples include:

- Detection of the Tay-Sachs gene in a carrier (see Chapter 16 for more information on Tay-Sachs disease)
- Elimination of paternity of an alleged father with 99% accuracy
- Detection of Down syndrome and neural tube defects in a fetus by testing the mother's blood (see Chapter 19 for more information about Down syndrome and neural tube defects)

Examining the Evidence

1. Why does a paternity test exclude an alleged father but not identify one directly?

_____

_____

_____

2. What are three advantages of knowing that a fetus has a disorder such as a neural tube defect or Down syndrome?

_____

_____

_____

Chapter **35** **Biotechnology Research and Development Careers**

3. Why do some people not want to have genetic testing done to determine any defects that might be present in a fetus?

_____

_____

_____

Cloning Controversy

Scientists at George Washington University cloned a human embryo in 1993. In this case, flawed embryos were divided and allowed to grow to the 32-cell stage. Embryos that contain 32 cells are often used for in vitro implantation. These cells were discarded after 6 days. No clear guidelines exist for this type of research and human experimentation. The American Fertility Society (AFS) has set voluntary guidelines that prohibit human embryos from being developed in a test tube longer than 14 days.

Examining the Evidence

1. What might be some concerns regarding the cloning of human embryos?

_____

_____

_____

2. What guidelines could be established to maintain an ethical policy regarding the cloning of human embryos?

_____

_____

_____

3. How can the public's perception of biotechnology research be improved?

_____

_____

_____

Exercises in Genetic Counseling

Consider the following situations that might occur in a genetic counseling center. Describe what action you feel would be appropriate for the counselor to follow.

Situation One

The patient comes in for testing to determine whether her fetus inherited two genes for cystic fibrosis. Testing is done on the woman and her husband. The blood tests show that the fetus does have the condition but that the husband is not a carrier. The woman forbids the counselor from telling the husband that the child is not his.

How would you respond if you were the genetic counselor?

_____

_____

_____

Situation Two

Two patients have the genetic condition polydactyly. They want their fetus tested for the condition. They inform the counselor of their intention to abort any fetus that is "normal," or without the condition. They feel that they do not want to raise a child who is different from them.

386

How would you respond if you were the genetic counselor?

_____

_____

_____

Situation Three

A patient carries the genetic trait for sickle cell anemia. She tells you that she will abort any fetus that carries the gene, because she wants the condition to end with her generation.

    How would you respond if you were the genetic counselor?

_____

_____

_____

INTERNET ACTIVITIES

Education and Career Research

Use the following links, other Internet resources, and information available by telephone or mail inquiry to determine the educational cost of one biotechnology career and the salary that might be earned in the local area. Use the information to complete Table 35-2.

Suggested Websites

Salary.com: http://salary.com
Monster.com: http://monster.com
Occupational Outlook Handbook: http://www.bls.gov/oco/
National Center for Biotechnology Information (NCBI): http://www.ncbi.nlm.nih.gov/

TABLE 35-2 Education and Career Research

CAREER	INSTITUTION FOR EDUCATION	COST OF EDUCATION	POTENTIAL EARNINGS

Chapter **35** **Biotechnology Research and Development Careers**